Behavioral Health
Protocols and Treatment Plans
for Recreational Therapy

Second Edition

Karen Grote, MS, CTRS
Sara Warner, MA, CTRS

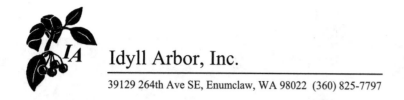

Idyll Arbor, Inc.

39129 264th Ave SE, Enumclaw, WA 98022 (360) 825-7797

Idyll Arbor, Inc. Editor: Thomas M. Blaschko

ISBN 9781882883929 paper
ISBN 9781611580259 ebook

All royalties from this book
will be donated to the
Recreational Therapy Foundation.

For more information about the Recreational Therapy Foundation,
please visit the website at
www.RecreationalTherapyFoundation.org.

Publisher's Note:

We have promoted the development and publishing of this book because we feel that those who use the services of a recreational therapist deserve the best possible care. This book was written for recreational therapy professionals (Certified Therapeutic Recreation Specialists) and for licensed recreational therapists.

To the best of our knowledge, the information and recommendations of this book reflect currently accepted practice. Nevertheless, they cannot be considered absolute and universal. Recommendations for therapy for a particular individual must be considered in light of the individual's needs and condition. The authors and publisher disclaim responsibility for any adverse effects resulting directly or indirectly from the suggested protocols or treatment plans, from any undetected errors, or from the reader's misunderstanding of the text.

Part 2 of this book includes sample individualized goals, objectives, and interventions that can be used in designing problem-centered interdisciplinary treatment plans for clients. This chapter was originally published independently as *Sample Treatment Plans for Therapeutic Recreation* (1990) by Karen Grote. There is a continuing need for competence in this area.

Contents

Contents

Contents

Acknowledgement

The authors would like to thank our friend and colleague, Bob Krider, for his advice and consultation in the development of this second edition.

Introduction

The first edition of this book was published in 1995 in an effort to help therapists respond to the growing requests for protocols, standardized treatment plans, and critical pathways. These new documents were meant to standardize care, define appropriate treatment, and in some way predict what outcome is expected from treatment.

One piece the reader will find missing from this edition is the section on critical pathways. Starting in the 1980s there was an emphasis on the development of critical pathways. First, they were used in post-surgical areas. Later their use spread to most other medical and surgical areas of medical centers. The intention was to develop a prescribed plan with interventions following a planned time frame. The pathways were supposed to increase efficiency, improve communication among staff, and increase desired patient outcomes. After years in practice there was a widespread lack of agreement on the impact of critical pathways on hospital resources and desired outcomes. Many of the pathways had limited effectiveness and did not decrease length of stay. Pathway utilization has not been a strong predictor of pathway effectiveness (Dy et al, 2005).

As a result, the authors have decided to delete the critical pathway section from this edition of the book and to, instead, offer the reader additional protocols. This edition contains six new or rewritten diagnostic protocols and eleven new or rewritten program protocols. Unique to this edition, there are diagnostic and program protocols specifically addressing the child/adolescent, the adult, and the geriatric populations. While these protocols only begin to address the breadth and scope of recreational therapy services, we believe they are a fair representation of typical practice, with a few surprising modalities included.

With the exception of the program protocols for My Life Collage and Octaband® Movement, all of the protocols included here were written by Certified Therapeutic Recreation Specialists (CTRSs). They are designed to be used by a CTRS or a licensed recreational therapist.

The therapist will find information on three elements of client treatment in this book: diagnostic protocols, program protocols, and symptom protocols (treatment plans). The therapist will be able to modify the contents of this book to fit both the needs of the clients and the needs of the facility.

Protocols

The first part of the book will acquaint the therapist with two different kinds of protocols — diagnostic and program protocols. Symptom protocols, also called treatment plans, will be covered in the second half of the book.

A *diagnostic protocol* identifies what treatment is offered to clients who have a specific diagnosis. For instance, it describe what modalities you use with a person who has a schizophrenic disorder. The idea behind diagnostic protocols is that most clients with a similar diagnosis should have similar needs. The recreational therapist draws upon the strength of the protocols to address the primary needs of the client diagnostic group. For the recreational therapist with a significant mix of client diagnoses these protocols may be problematic because the psychosocial deficiencies and needs demonstrated by one client may be significantly different from other clients on the same unit. These protocols may also be called teaching protocols.

A *program protocol* describes each program that is offered. Programs may include just one or two related activities (stretching and cardiovascular activity) or they may include unlimited activity choices (paper crafts to enhance expression). The unifying element is that all the activities selected will help the client move toward the desired outcome. Program protocols should include structure, process, and outcome criteria. They should also consider referral considerations, contraindications, risk management issues, and any specific personnel training or certification requirement (e.g., a Water Safety Instructor certification).

The third type of protocol may be called a *symptom protocol*, but is otherwise known as a treatment plan. This type of protocol is written to describe appropriate treatment offered in response to very specific symptomatology displayed by the client. These may also be referred to as functionally based protocols. The last section of this book contains treatment plans based on symptomatology.

Table 1: Examples of Protocols

Type of Protocol	Example of Protocol
Diagnostic	Depression
Program	Aquatics
Symptom (Treatment Plan)	Uncontrolled anger outbursts

There are many forces that contribute to the need for development of all three kinds of protocols in recreational therapy. Health care organizations are concerned with providing the best quality of care, with the most efficacious outcomes for the clients, in the most cost-effective way. These drive the current effort to base health care treatment on efficacy-based research. In recreational therapy, protocols can also be used as training modules to moderate the effect of geographic variation in academic training and clinical practice, and to further establish a research-supported body of common practice.

Recreational therapists who work in rehabilitation settings were the first who were asked to write protocols, or standards of accepted care for the different diagnostic groups that they treat. The word protocol was used in several different contexts, often without any consensus across professions.

In the recreational therapy literature, several authors have discussed protocol development. Knight and Johnson (1989) wrote that "protocols are a group of strategies or actions initiated in response to a problem, an issue, or a symptom of a client." Olsson (1990) defined a protocol as "a set of very specific instructions, regulations and requirements that govern an agency's recreational therapy practice and when implemented produce specific treatment outcomes." Ferguson (1991) further added, "Protocols provide information detailing the specific problem or need to be addressed and provide a set of expected outcomes which can be measured and examined."

Stumbo & Peterson (2009) define an outcome-oriented intervention as being:

- Focused on a systematic assessment of client characteristics, needs, and/or deficits
- Designed in advance to be efficient and effective in its delivery
- Able to produce targeted, meaningful, timely, and desired client outcomes
- Able to produce evaluation data indicating achievement (or non-achievement) of client outcomes
- Part of a larger systematic, comprehensive set of quality programs

The *Standards for the Practice of Therapeutic Recreation* (ATRA, 2000) identifies a written plan of operation, along with treatment protocols, as a necessary feature of a therapeutic recreation program. The treatment protocols serve as a map for therapists on how to provide successful treatment for their clients.

A protocol may be compared to a city map. It outlines which city streets the client will be taking, and maybe even which gas stations or bus stops will be used on the way from "Point A" to "Point B." The therapist would work with the treatment team and the client to select the best combination of protocols (e.g., relaxation techniques, cooking skills, social etiquette) for the client to achieve the desired outcome at the end of treatment.

Protocols are written plans which outline:

- Who is to take part in treatment
- What specific treatment will be offered
- What outcomes the client should see as a result of the treatment

Departments need to design diagnostic protocols of standardized care procedures for frequently treated diagnostic groups. This step is important for establishing a common practice among therapists who work in a department, so that clients can know what treatment outcomes they can expect in the program regardless of which therapist is assigned to treat them. Other professionals can also come to depend on the standardized delivery of services. These protocols include assessment criteria for the client, a review of symptoms from the current edition of the *Diagnostic and Statistical Manual of Mental Disorders, Fourth Edition, Text Revision (DSM-IV-TR),* process criteria to identify the particular programs that will be suitable in the treatment of this diagnosis, and outcome criteria to identify the anticipated achievable goals from participation in this treatment.

An important element of the protocols featured in this book is the criteria used. *Structure* criteria describe the way the group or program is organized and what modalities will be used. *Process* criteria describe what methods the therapist will employ to facilitate the modalities, including perhaps what approach the therapist will use, how much assistance will be provided, or what instruction will be provided. *Outcome* criteria list what benefits the client can expect from participation in the program.

Other Types of Protocols in Health Care

Smith-Marker (1988) looked at protocols in a different way in the nursing literature and identified three types: independent, collaborative, and interdependent protocols. Independent protocols were discipline specific, collaborative were written by two disciplines that would co-treat or team-treat clients with common modalities, and the interdependent protocols were interdisciplinary and required a physician's order to initiate treatment for a given client.

Physicians design agency-specific diagnostic protocols. These protocols identify the known etiology and symptomatology as outlined in the current *DSM-IV-TR,* the accepted treatment practices among that group of physicians, and the expected outcomes when following this protocol.

Protocols, no matter which kind, should be well thought out and based on both the therapist's clinical experience and on the experience and research of others. Whenever possible, diagnostic and program protocols for recreational therapy should be annotated with outcome findings from efficacy-based research. It is critical in our field that we continue to support and conduct research to identify appropriate interventions which achieve expected outcomes.

Diagnostic Protocols

A diagnostic protocol is an outline of the treatment and services routinely provided to clients with a specific diagnosis. The protocol is defined by an outline with six parts:

1. Diagnostic category
2. Assessment criteria
3. Symptoms typically observed
4. Process criteria
5. Outcome criteria
6. Bibliography of supporting literature

In behavioral health settings the diagnoses will be described in the most current edition of the *Diagnostic and Statistical Manual of Mental Disorders* (currently the *DSM-IV-TR*). This makes up the first part of the diagnostic protocol outline.

The second part of the protocol outline contains the types of assessments the therapist will complete prior to "admitting" a client to that particular protocol. The therapist will select the most appropriate internal or standardized forms for assessing the client based on the guidance in the protocol, the facility's expectations, and the therapist's clinical judgment. The assessment establishes a baseline which can be used to measure changes in the client as treatment progresses.

It is important that the therapist make some determination about the client's status before initiating the diagnostic protocol. There may be clients who have been given a particular diagnosis but who are inappropriate for inclusion in all elements of the protocol. For example, a client may be diagnosed with a major depressive episode and have a secondary diagnosis of dementia. While the client may benefit from some of the treatment modalities, her ability to grasp more didactic elements of the protocol may be limited.

The symptom list is also available in the *DSM-IV-TR*. The therapist will want to identify symptoms from the *DSM-IV-TR* which are responsive to recreational therapy intervention and which relate to the client's ability to have a functional leisure lifestyle. There may also be symptoms which are common within the diagnostic group and which impact the client's ability to perform other advanced activities of daily living.

The process criteria refer to the steps taken and services provided by the therapist to complete the protocol and effective treatment. This part leads the therapists from inception to completion of the protocol. The process criteria should be written in such a way that consistency among therapists is assured.

Outcome criteria are the measurable changes brought about for the client as a direct result of participation in the protocol. With each program or service in the process criteria, there should be a positive benefit anticipated as a direct result in the outcome criteria.

Finally, the diagnostic protocol outline includes a bibliography of books, articles, and other professional literature, which supports the efficacy of the treatment or service provided. References which help identify specific needs and characteristics of clients within a diagnostic group should also be listed.

The following page shows a sample format for diagnostic protocols. The examples in this section include many of the major mental illnesses for adult and geriatric behavioral health clients and the addition of diagnoses that are typically seen in child and/or adolescent settings. The therapist is encouraged to use them as a framework for developing an agency-specific set of diagnostic protocols, or they may be modified to reflect the facility's system of treatment delivery. You may also find that the diagnostic protocols need to be updated periodically to keep up with client variations and growing scientific data in efficacy-based research.

Sample Diagnostic Protocol Format

I.   Diagnosis

State the specific diagnostic group from the current edition of the *Diagnostic and Statistical Book for Mental Disorders (DSM-IV-TR)*.

II.   Assessment Criteria

Identify how the client with this diagnosis will be assessed, what information will be gathered, and what standardized assessment should be used.

III.   Symptoms

List the cluster of psychiatric symptoms that are used to accurately diagnose a client with this disorder. Add any additional common psychosocial symptoms that recreational therapy interventions are reasonably able to treat.

IV.   Process Criteria

Identify the steps the therapist will take to assess and treat this type of client. Consider all relevant and appropriate modalities that will be used in the treatment plan.

V.   Outcome Criteria

State the outcomes the client can expect after s/he is treated by a recreational therapist who employs this protocol.

VI.   Bibliography

Record the bibliographical references used to develop this protocol.

Attention Deficit/Hyperactivity Disorder

I. Diagnosis

Attention Deficit/Hyperactivity Disorder

II. Assessment Criteria

In a clinical setting, a client may be assessed by a psychiatrist or psychologist using a thorough history which should include detailed information about the child's behavior, environment, school, and medical records. In addition, observations in various settings will also be completed. After the agency's screening assessment, the recreational therapist may find the Comprehensive Evaluation in Recreational Therapy (CERT-Psych) useful in a clinical setting to assess and monitor inattention and hyperactive behaviors among clients with Attention Deficit/Hyperactivity Disorder symptoms. Other assessments of leisure interests and functioning may include Leisure Interest Measure (LIM), Teen Leisurescope Plus, or the Therapeutic Recreation Activity Assessment.

III. Symptoms

The symptoms of Attention Deficit/Hyperactivity Disorder may be demonstrated through many kinds of inattention which include:

1. Not paying attention to details
2. Making careless mistakes
3. Messy work
4. Difficulty sustaining attention
5. Not seeming to listen
6. Not following through on instructions or tasks
7. Difficulty organizing tasks
8. Not engaging in mental tasks
9. Losing things
10. Easily distracted
11. Forgetfulness
12. Frequent shifts in conversations

In addition, such a client will exhibit symptoms of hyperactivity and impulsivity:

1. Fidgety
2. Leaving seat frequently
3. Running about excessively
4. Difficulty engaging in quiet play
5. Often "on the go"
6. Talking excessively
7. Unnecessarily making noise
8. Blurting out

9. Impatience
10. Difficulty waiting for turn
11. Interrupting or intruding

This type of client may also experience:

1. Low self-esteem
2. Poor frustration tolerance
3. Mood lability
4. Excessive gross motor activity
5. Non-assertive social skills
6. Academic problems

IV. Process Criteria

The primary goals of treatment for individuals with Attention Deficit/Hyperactivity Disorder are to increase attention span, decrease hyperactivity and impulsivity, and improve pro-social skills. Pro-social skills include basic communication skills, as well as expressing strong emotions, resolving conflicts, using negotiation techniques, communicating needs, and showing empathy for others in an appropriate manner.

The recreational therapist develops an individualized treatment plan based on the symptoms that the client presents. While the treatment modalities are important to treat the client, the techniques the therapist uses for improvement are also important. Behavior modification techniques have been proven to be extremely helpful with clients who are diagnosed with Attention Deficit/Hyperactivity Disorder. Through behavior modification, the therapist works to replace the client's negative behaviors with more desirable ones by utilizing reinforcement. For example, if a client is having a difficult time sharing supplies, the recreational therapist may give the client a gold star on his/her chart each time s/he shares without prompting or becoming argumentative.

Clients with Attention Deficit/Hyperactivity Disorder will benefit from the use of modalities that encourage following directions, social interactions with peers, and regulating hyperactivity or impulsivity such as:

1. Pet assisted therapy
2. Games
3. Therapeutic art
4. Drama
5. Exercise
6. Structured tasks
7. Socialization activities

Psychoeducational groups about social and assertiveness training, stress management, and leisure education can be helpful if the client is able to process the information and gain some awareness. These may need to be conducted in individual treatment if the client is overly hyper or impulsive during the group process.

The recreational therapist should also inquire about the client's behavior in a variety of situations and settings because signs of the disorder may be minimal or absent when the person is under very strict control, engaged in especially interesting activities, in a one-on-one situation, or while the person experiences frequent rewards for appropriate behavior.

V.   Outcome Criteria

At the completion of treatment the client will be able to:

1. Demonstrate the ability to follow instructions
2. Improve concentration and decision-making
3. Successfully complete a project or task without becoming distracted
4. Demonstrate increased knowledge and skills in social interactions
5. Exhibit improved communication skills
6. Demonstrate appropriate social etiquette
7. Demonstrate increased self-regulation ability
8. Identify a plan for effective stress reduction
9. Report awareness of the benefits of leisure participation
10. Identify a personal leisure plan for use after discharge

VI. Bibliography

American Psychiatric Association. (2000). *Diagnostic and Statistical Manual of Mental Disorders (Fourth Edition, Text Revision)*. Washington, DC.

Attention Deficit/Hyperactivity Disorder (ADHD). http://www.nimh.nih.gov/health/publications/attention-deficit-hyperactivity-disorder/adhd_booklet.pdf. National Institute of Mental Health. Retrieved 11-3-11.

Behavior Modification. http://www.healthline.com/galecontent/behavioral-therapy. Retrieved 11-3-11.

Coyle, C., Riley, R., & Shank, J. (eds.) (1991). *Benefits of Therapeutic Recreation: A Consensus View*. Ravensdale, WA: Idyll Arbor, Inc.

Kaufman, G., & Raphael, L. (1990). *Stick Up for Yourself! Every Kid's Guide to Personal Power and Positive Self-Esteem*. Minneapolis: Free Spirit Publishing.

Kaufman, G., & Raphael, L. (1991). *Teacher's Guide to Stick Up for Yourself! A 10 Part Course In Self-Esteem and Assertiveness for Kids*. Minneapolis: Free Spirit Publishing.

Korb, K. L., Azok, S. D., & Leutenberg, E. A. (1992). *SEALS + Plus: Self-Esteem and Life Skills: Reproducible Activity-Based Handouts Created for Teachers and Counselors*. Beachwood, OH: Wellness Reproductions.

Peer Functioning in Children with ADHD. http://jpepsy.oxfordjournals.org/content/32/6/655.full.pdf+html Retrieved 11-3-11.

Oppositional Defiant Disorder

I. Diagnosis

Oppositional Defiant Disorder

II. Assessment Criteria

In a clinical setting, a client may be assessed by a psychiatrist or psychologist using a thorough psychological history, clinical observation, or the use of standardized tests. The recreational therapist may use the agency's screening tool. The Comprehensive Evaluation in Recreational Therapy (CERT-Psych) may also be useful in a clinical setting to monitor defiant and disobedient behaviors among clients with Oppositional Defiant Disorder symptoms. Other assessments of leisure interests and functioning may include Leisure Interest Measure (LIM), Leisure Attitude Measure (LAM), Leisure Satisfaction Measure (LSM), or Teen Leisurescope Plus.

III. Symptoms

The symptoms of Oppositional Defiant Disorder may be demonstrated through many kinds of disobedient behavior including the following symptoms:

1. Resistant to following directions
2. Limit testing
3. Persistently stubborn
4. Hostile or argumentative towards authority figures
5. Losing his or her temper frequently
6. Deliberately annoying people
7. Blaming others for his/her mistakes or misbehaviors
8. Easily annoyed by others
9. Unwilling to compromise
10. Angry and resentful
11. Spiteful and vindictive
12. Verbally aggressive

IV. Process Criteria

The primary goals of treatment for individuals with Oppositional Defiant Disorder are to decrease defiant and disobedient behaviors, improve the client's prosocial skills, and to control frustration and anger.

The recreational therapist develops an individualized treatment plan based on the symptoms that the client presents. While the treatment modalities are important to treat the individual, the attitude which the therapist utilizes to approach the actual treatment is also critical in the process of improvement. Clients with Oppositional Defiant Disorder often argue with adults and authority figures, so it is important the therapist avoids power struggles. For example, if you ask the individual to take a time out in the hallway due to disruptive behavior and s/he begins to argue simply state "Your time will begin when you are seated in the hallway" instead of adding additional time.

Clients with Oppositional Defiant Disorder will benefit from the use of modalities that encourage following directions, social interactions with peers, and regulating frustration or anger such as:

1. Games
2. Therapeutic art
3. Gardening
4. Structured tasks
5. Social interaction

Psychoeducational groups about anger management, assertiveness training, and problem solving can be helpful if the client is able to process the information and gain some awareness. These may need to be conducted in individual treatment if the client is overly disobedient during the group process.

Clients with Oppositional Defiant Disorder tend not to comply with treatment protocols, so additional mechanisms designed to enhance compliance and completion of treatment protocols should be used. For example, utilizing a reward system may keep a client motivated to continue to work on treatment goals.

V.   Outcome Criteria

At the completion of treatment the client will be able to:

1. Demonstrate improved ability to follow instructions
2. Engage in discussions without becoming argumentative or defiant
3. Demonstrate increased knowledge and skills in social interactions
4. Exhibit improved communication skills
5. Report reduced agitation, frustration, and anger
6. Demonstrate self-regulation ability
7. Identify and utilize various coping skills independently
8. Demonstrate ability to take responsibility for decisions or mistakes

VI. Bibliography

American Psychiatric Association. (2000). *Diagnostic and Statistical Manual of Mental Disorders (Fourth Edition, Text Revision)*. Washington, DC.

Burke, J. D., Loeber, R., & Birmaher, B. (2004). Oppositional defiant disorder and conduct disorder: A review of the past 10 years, Part II. *Focus: The Journal of Lifelong Learning in Psychiatry, Volume II*(4), 558-576.

Facts for Families of Children with Oppositional Defiant Disorder. http://www.aacap.org/cs/root/facts_for_families/children_with_oppositional_defiant_disorder. American Academy of Child and Adolescent Psychiatry. Retrieved 12-11-11.

Reactive Attachment Disorder, Inhibited Type

I. Diagnosis

Reactive Attachment Disorder, Inhibited Type

II. Assessment Criteria

In a clinical setting, a mental health professional must first determine if the client has one of the following in his/her history: disregard of the child's basic emotional needs for comfort, stimulation, and attention; disregard for the child's basic physical needs; or repeated change in the primary caregiver that prevented formation of stable attachments. Such a client may then be assessed by a psychiatrist or psychologist using a variety of sources including general observations, interviews, standardized questionnaires, an assessment of social cognition, and a comprehensive psychiatric examination. The recreational therapist may use the facility's screening assessment or choose from other standardized tools in the field. The Comprehensive Evaluation in Recreational Therapy (CERT-Psych) or The Functional Assessment of Characteristics for Therapeutic Recreation, Revised (FACTR-R) can be helpful in a clinical setting to assess and monitor social relatedness among clients with Reactive Attachment Disorder, Inhibited Type symptoms. Other assessments of leisure interests and functioning may include Leisure Interest Measure (LIM), Leisure Motivation Scale (LMS), Leisure Attitude Measure (LAM), or Teen Leisurescope Plus.

III. Symptoms

The symptoms of Reactive Attachment Disorder, Inhibited Type may be demonstrated through many kinds of developmentally inappropriate social relatedness including the following symptoms:

1. Fails to initiate or respond to most social interactions
2. Excessively introverted
3. Extremely watchful
4. Exceptionally hesitant responses

This type of client may also experience:

1. A dislike of physical touch
2. Low self-esteem
3. An inability to express emotions
4. Difficulty forming meaningful relationships
5. Distrust of others
6. Anger or frustration
7. Need to be in control
8. An undeveloped conscience

IV. Process Criteria

The primary goals of treatment for individuals with Reactive Attachment Disorder, Inhibited Type are to help the client learn how to interact in social settings, increase self-esteem, and to learn how to express himself/herself in a healthy manner.

The recreational therapist develops an individualized treatment plan based on the symptoms that the client presents. Clients with Reactive Attachment Disorder, Inhibited Type will benefit from the use of modalities that encourage social interactions, give an opportunity for self-expression, and provide the chance to accomplish or succeed in a task, such as:

1. Pet assisted therapy
2. Equine therapy
3. Therapeutic art
4. Creative expression
5. Social interaction
6. Team games

Psychoeducational groups about social and assertiveness training and stress management can be helpful if the client is able to process the information and gain some awareness.

V. Outcome Criteria

At the completion of treatment the client will be able to:

1. Demonstrate increased knowledge and skills in social interactions
2. Increase frequency of peer interactions
3. Demonstrate ability to initiate social interactions
4. Report improved self-confidence
5. Demonstrate the ability to express thoughts and feelings

VI. Bibliography

American Psychiatric Association. (2000). *Diagnostic and Statistical Manual of Mental Disorders (Fourth Edition, Text Revision)*. Washington, DC.

Attachment and Reactive Attachment Disorders.
http://helpguide.org/mental/parenting_bonding_reactive_attachment_disorder.htm. Retrieved 11-15-11.

Best practices in Children's Mental Health.
http://kuscholarworks.ku.edu/dspace/bitstream/1808/3879/1/bestpracticesreport11.pdf. Retrieved: 11-15-11.

Major Depressive Episode

I.   Diagnosis

Major Depressive Episode

II. Assessment Criteria

The assessment includes an evaluation of the client's cognitive, social, and physical functioning, including the client's motivation, leisure interests, and patterns of participation. The agency's screening assessment may be followed by administering the Leisure Motivation Scale, the Leisure Attitude Measurement, the Leisure Satisfaction Measurement, the Leisure Competence Measure, the Leisure Diagnostic Battery, the Leisure Interest Measurement, the Free-Time Boredom Measure, and/or the Teen or Adult Leisurescope Plus, as indicated.

III. Symptoms

A client diagnosed with major depression will experience five or more of the following symptoms:

1. Depressed mood for at least two weeks for adults, or four weeks for teens
2. Diminished interest or pleasure
3. Significant weight loss or gain
4. Insomnia or hypersomnia
5. Psychomotor agitation or retardation
6. Fatigue or loss of energy
7. Feelings of worthlessness or inappropriate guilt
8. Difficulty concentrating or making decisions
9. Recurrent thoughts of death, up to and including planning and executing suicide

In addition, such a client may also exhibit:

1. A lack of initiative for usual activities
2. Diminished social interaction
3. Inadequate assertive social skills
4. Lack of energy
5. Ruminating thoughts
6. Cognitive distortions

IV. Process Criteria

The recreational therapist develops an individualized treatment plan, considering all subjective and objective assessment information, and provides treatment to the client from among the following modalities:

1. Exercise
2. Stress management and relaxation therapy
3. Leisure education

4. Friendship development
5. Structured tasks
6. Assertiveness training
7. Journaling

V. Outcome Criteria

At the completion of treatment the client will be able to:

1. Report increased level of energy
2. Demonstrate increased self-regulation ability
3. Identify a plan to use effective stress reducers
4. Report awareness of benefits of leisure participation
5. Identify a personal leisure plan for use after discharge
6. Identify strategies for increasing social supports
7. Demonstrate increased social initiative
8. Demonstrate improved concentration and decision-making
9. Demonstrate assertive communication style
10. Report a decrease in ruminating thoughts

VI. Bibliography

American Psychiatric Association. (2000). *Diagnostic and Statistical Manual of Mental Disorders (Fourth Edition, Text Revision)*. Washington, DC.

Berger, B. G. (1983). Stress reduction through exercise: The mind-body connection. *Motor Skills: Theory into Practice, 7*, 31-46.

Carruthers, C. & Hood, C. (2002). Coping skills program for individuals with alcoholism. *Therapeutic Recreation Journal, 36*(2), 154-171.

Compton, D. M. & Iso-Ahola, S. E. (Eds.) (1994). *Leisure and Mental Health*. Park City, UT: Family Development Resources, Inc.

Coyle, C. P., Kinney, W. B., Riley, B., & Shank, J. W. (1991). *Benefits of Therapeutic Recreation: A Consensus View*. Ravensdale, WA: Idyll Arbor, Inc.

Dehn, D. (1995). *Leisure Step Up*. Ravensdale, WA: Idyll Arbor, Inc.

Eisler, R. M., Hersen, M., & Miller, P. M. (1974). Shaping components of assertive behavior with instruction and feedback. *American Journal of Psychiatry, 131*, 1344-1347.

Epperson, A., Witt, P.A., & Hitzhusen, G. (1977). *Leisure Counseling: An Aspect of Leisure Education*. Springfield: Charles C. Thomas.

Gortner, E., Rude, S., Pennebaker, J. (2006). Benefits of expressive writing in lowering rumination and depressive symptoms. *Behavioral Therapy, 37*, 292-303.

Grossman, A. H. (1976). Power of activity in a treatment setting. *Therapeutic Recreation Journal, 10* (4), 119-124.

Grossman P., Niemann, L., Schmidt, S., & Walach, H. (2004). Mindfulness-based stress reduction and health benefits: A meta-analysis. *Journal of Psychosomatic Research, 57*, 35-43.

Harrist, S., Carlozzi, B., McGovern, A. & Harrist, A. (2007). Benefits of expressive writing and expressive talking about life goals. *Journal of Research in Personality, 41*, 923-930.

Horowitz, S. (2008). Evidence-based health outcomes of expressive writing. *Alternative and Complimentary Therapies, 14*, 194-198.

Iwasaki, Y., Coyle, C., Shank, J., Salzer, M., Baron, D., Messina, E., Mitchell, L., Ryan, A., Koons, G., & Kishbauch, G. (2010). Exploring the role of leisure in recovery from mental illness. Abstracts from the 2010 American Therapeutic Recreation Association, 21-26.

Jacobs, G. (2001). The physiology of mind-body interactions: The stress response and the relaxation response. *The Journal of Alternative and Complimentary Medicine. 7*(Supp 1), S83-S92.

Jorm, A., Morgan, A. & Hetrick, S. (2008). Relaxation for depression. Cochrane Database of Systematic Reviews 4, CD007142. DOI: 10.1002/14651858.CD007142.pub2.

McGlynn, G. (1987). *Dynamics of Fitness: A Practical Approach*. Dubuque, IA: Wm. C. Brown.

Morgan, W. P. & Goldston, S. E. (1987). *Exercise and Mental Health*. Washington, DC: Hemisphere Publishing.

Russonello, C., O'Brien, K., & Parks, J. (2009). The effectiveness of casual video games in improving mood and decreasing stress. *Journal of CyberTherapy and Rehabilitation, 2*(1), 53-66.

Bipolar Disorder, Mania

I. Diagnosis

Bipolar Disorder, Mania

II. Assessment Criteria

In a clinical setting, a client may be assessed by a psychiatrist or psychologist using a good history, clinical observation, medical testing, or the use of standardized tests. The recreational therapist may find the Psychogeriatric Dependency Rating Scale useful in a geriatric setting to assess and monitor disruptive behaviors among clients with manic symptoms. The Quality of Life Enjoyment & Satisfaction Questionnaire (Q-LES-Q) is a self-administered questionnaire that includes subscales that assess functioning in physical health, subjective feelings, leisure-time activities, social relationships, and general activities. Other assessments of leisure interests and functioning may include the Leisure Interest Survey (CompuTR), Comprehensive Evaluation in Recreational Therapy (CERT-Psych), or the Leisurescope Plus.

III. Symptoms

The symptoms of mania may be demonstrated through many kinds of excessive behavior, including the following:

1. Increased energy
2. Unusual talkativeness
3. Hyperactivity
4. Racing thoughts
5. Distractibility
6. Irritability
7. Little need for sleep
8. Inflated self-esteem
9. Grandiose thoughts about one's abilities
10. Hyper-excitability
11. Euphoria
12. Hyper-vigilance, perhaps being awake for several days

In addition, a person with mania may engage in risky and reckless behaviors that would normally be out of character, including:

1. Spending sprees
2. Unprotected sexual encounters
3. Binge drinking or use of drugs
4. Making rash financial decisions or foolish investments

IV. Process Criteria

The primary goals of treatment of individuals with mania are to decrease the disruptive behaviors, improve concentration, and increase knowledge and insight about the manic symptoms.

The recreational therapist develops an individualized treatment plan based on the symptoms that the client presents. The therapist uses not only modalities (activities) to treat the client. The attitude that the therapist uses to intervene is critical in the process of improvement. Clients with mania can elicit negative or reactionary responses from caregivers and it is important to have a clear understanding of this potential process.

It is also true that clients with mania may become overstimulated by some activities or social environments. Many times the specific modality becomes less critical in treatment than the feedback and limit-setting given by the therapist to the client about his/her behavior. It is always best to treat the symptoms as they appear. For instance, when a client is very agitated, not participating in a certain modality may be the best treatment. (See the section on Treatment Plans for further suggestions about attitudinal interventions for disruptive behaviors.) Individual treatment may be provided if the client is disruptive to the group process through hyper-talkativeness or frequent interruptions. Clients who are taught cognitive behavioral therapy can learn to recognize and discuss their moods, then change their thinking about them.

Clients with mania will benefit from the use of modalities that encourage concentration, following directions, and moderating behavior such as:

1. Exercise
2. Games
3. Art expression
4. Gardening
5. Stress reduction and relaxation techniques and/or meditation
6. Good sleeping hygiene
7. Anxiety reduction
8. Cognitive behavioral therapy

V. Outcome Criteria

At the completion of treatment, the client may expect to:

1. Conduct conversation without disruptive behaviors
2. Report a reduction in anxiety
3. Reduce disruptive behaviors
4. Improve concentration and the ability to follow directions
5. Be able to describe how built-up stress may trigger a manic episode
6. Create a personal plan to manage stress
7. Be able to use relaxation techniques and/or meditation independently
8. Feel more emotional control

VI. Bibliography

American Psychiatric Association. (2000). *Diagnostic and Statistical Manual of Mental Disorders (Fourth Edition, Text Revision)*. Washington, DC.

AstraZeneca Pharmaceuticals (2004). *Manual of Rating Scales for the Assessment of Mood Disorder*. Wilmington, DE.

burlingame, j. & Blaschko, T. M. (2010). *Assessment Tools for Recreational Therapy, 4th Ed*. Enumclaw, WA. Idyll Arbor, Inc.

Endicott, J., Nee, J., Harrison, W. et al. (1993). Quality of life enjoyment and satisfaction questionnaire: A new scale. *Psychopharmacology Bulletin, 29*, 321-326.

Healthline: Bipolar overview. www.healthline.com/health/bipolar-disorder-overview. Retrieved 12/14/11.

Healthline: Bipolar disorder symptoms. www.healthline.com/health/bipolar-disorder-symptoms. Retrieved 12/14/11.

Healthline: It may be possible to predict mood swings: Study. www.healthline.com/healthday/it-may-be-possible-to-predict-bipolar-mood-swings-study. Retrieved 12/14/11.

Miklowitz, D. (2011). Functional impairment, stress, and psychological intervention in bipolar disorder. *Current Psychiatry Reports, 13*(6), 504-512.

Mullen, J., Endicott, J., Hirshfeld, R., Yonkers, K., Targum, S., & Bullinger, A. (2004). *Manual of Rating Scales for the Assessment of Mood Disorders*. Wilmington, DE: Astra Zeneca Pharmaceuticals LP.

Vieta, E., Pacchiarotti, I., Scott, J., Sanchez-Moreno, J., Di Marzo, S., & Colom, F. (2005). Evidence based research on the efficacy of psychologic interventions in bipolar disorders: A critical review. *Current Psychiatry Reports, 7*(6), 449-455.

Vieta, E., Pacchiarotti, I., Valenti, M., Berk, M., Scott, J., & Colom, F. (2009). A critical update on psychological interventions for bipolar disorder. *Current Psychiatry Reports, 11*(6), 494-502.

Schizophrenia and Other Psychotic Disorders

I. Diagnosis

Schizophrenia and Other Psychotic Disorders

II. Assessment Criteria

The assessment includes an evaluation of the client's cognitive, social, and physical functioning, and also the client's motivation, leisure skills and interests, and patterns of participation. Individuals with schizophrenia may display dysfunctional social relationships and lack leisure interests or the ability to execute a satisfying and healthy leisure lifestyle. The agency's screening assessment may be followed by the use of the Comprehensive Evaluation in Recreational Therapy (CERT-Psych), Leisure Motivation Scale, Leisure Interest Measurement, Leisure Attitude Measurement, and Leisurescope Plus, as indicated.

III. Symptoms

Symptoms typically include:

1. Delusions
2. Hallucinations
3. Disorganized thoughts
4. Grossly disorganized or catatonic behavior

Also, "negative" symptoms include:

1. Affect flattening
2. Diminished capacity for logical thinking
3. Lack of motivation

Clients with these disorders may also experience social and occupational dysfunction, concurrent mood disorders, or substance abuse.

IV. Process Criteria

The recreational therapist will develop an individualized treatment plan, considering all subjective and objective information, and provide treatment to the client from among the following modalities:

1. Exercise
2. Stress management
3. Leisure education
4. Friendship development
5. Structured tasks
6. Assertiveness training

V. Outcome Criteria

At the completion of treatment the client will be able to:

1. Sustain focus with active participation

2. Report increased level of energy

3. Identify and practice techniques to distract from symptoms of hallucinations and delusions

4. Identify a plan to use effective stress/symptom reducers after discharge

5. Report awareness of benefits of leisure participation

6. Identify a personal leisure plan for use after discharge

7. Identify strategies for increasing social supports

8. Demonstrate increased social initiative

9. Demonstrate improved concentration, decision-making, and follow-through

10. Demonstrate assertive communication style

VI. Bibliography

American Psychiatric Association. (2000). *Diagnostic and Statistical Manual of Mental Disorders (Fourth Edition, Text Revision)*. Washington, DC.

Ascher-Svanum, H. & Krause, A. A. (1991). *Psychoeducational Groups for Clients with Schizophrenia: A Guide for Practitioners*. Rockville: Aspen Publications.

Berger, B. G. (1983). Stress reduction through exercise: The mind-body connection. *Motor Skills: Theory Into Practice, 7*, 31-46.

Compton, D. M. & Iso-Ahola, S. E. (Eds.) (1994). *Leisure and Mental Health*. Park City, UT: Family Development Resources, Inc.

Coyle, C. P., Kinney, W. B., Riley, B., & Shank, J. W. (1991). *Benefits of Therapeutic Recreation: A Consensus View*. Ravensdale, WA: Idyll Arbor, Inc.

Dehn, D. (1995). *Leisure Step Up*. Ravensdale, WA: Idyll Arbor, Inc.

Eisler, R. M., Hersen, M., & Miller, P. M. (1974). Shaping components of assertive behavior with instruction and feedback. *American Journal of Psychiatry. 131*, 1344-1347.

Epperson, A., Witt, P.A., & Hitzhusen, G. (1977). *Leisure Counseling: An Aspect of Leisure Education*. Springfield: Charles C. Thomas.

Grossman, A. H. (1976). Power of activity in a treatment setting. *Therapeutic Recreation Journal. 10*(4), 119-124.

McGlynn, G. (1987). *Dynamics of Fitness: A Practical Approach*. Dubuque, IA: Wm. C. Brown.

Morgan, W. P. & Goldston, S. E. (1987). *Exercise and Mental Health*. Washington, DC Hemisphere Publishing.

Anxiety Disorders

I. Diagnosis

Anxiety Disorders

There are a number of anxiety disorders that may stand alone or be associated with a mood disorder. While anxiety is a normal human emotion and is supposed to keep us on our toes for an upcoming event, this normal anxiety should diminish when the event is over. Anxiety can interfere over time with one's occupational, social, and leisure functioning.

Generalized Anxiety Disorder (GAD) is diagnosed in clients who have a persistent feeling of dread and are anxious all the time, perhaps without knowing why. Their symptoms may be accompanied by insomnia, gastro-intestinal symptoms, restlessness, hopelessness, or fatigue.

Obsessive-Compulsive Disorder (OCD) is characterized by persistent, ruminating thoughts and compulsive behaviors, and repetitive patterns such as frequent hand washing, counting by sevens, checking and rechecking.

Post Traumatic Stress Disorder (PTSD) was first widely used as a diagnosis during the Vietnam era as soldiers were returning from war, but it is used more widely today to pertain to people who have been through a life-threatening situation from which they have a hard time moving on. The chief symptoms are nightmares and flashbacks which are more than a distant memory. It is as if the original event is occurring once again and all of the original negative emotion of fear or anxiety comes flooding back. Clients with PTSD usually also have mood disorders. They have a quick startle reflex and can be hypervigilant.

Anxiety Attacks or *Panic Disorder* refers to sudden, unexpected attacks of intense fear and anxiety. The physical symptoms such as a pounding heart, sweating, and hyperventilating can be distressing and mimic a heart attack. The client may or may not be able to determine the precipitant for the attacks.

II. Assessment Criteria

The assessment process will assist the therapist in determining how the anxiety disorder affects the social, physical, and leisure functioning of the client. The self-administered Psychological General Well-Being Index provides useful information about anxiety, depressed mood, positive well-being, self-control, general health, and vitality. Leisure functioning may also be assessed using the Leisure Motivation Scale (LMS), the Leisure Attitude Measurement (LAM), the Leisure Satisfaction Measure (LSM), or the Leisure Competence Measure (LCM).

III. Symptoms

The symptoms of anxiety disorders may include:

1. Feelings of dread
2. Trouble concentrating
3. Feeling tense and jumpy
4. Anticipating the worst
5. Irritability
6. Restlessness

7. Muscle tension, tremors or twitches, feeling shaky
8. Vague physical complaints
9. Avoidance of social situations and withdrawal
10. Increased heart rate
11. Trouble breathing, hyperventilation
12. Sweating
13. Feeling of losing control
14. Fear of passing out

IV. Process Criteria

There are many modalities that can be used to treat clients who have anxiety disorders. Some of these like exercise and relaxation techniques are designed to reduce muscular and nervous tension. Mindfulness-Based Cognitive Therapy is designed to assist the client to recognize, monitor, and regulate changing mood states. Still other modalities of recreational activities use the value of distraction to increase concentration and decrease ruminating thoughts. Finally, since the development of insight may actually reduce anxiety, clients may be encouraged to use expressive media like journaling, art expression, or creating collages.

These modalities will be encouraged for clients with anxiety disorders:

1. Exercise
2. Structured recreational activities
3. Expressive media — journaling, art expression, making collages
4. Mindfulness-Based Cognitive Therapy
5. Stress management
6. Relaxation techniques
7. Mindfulness meditation

V. Outcome Criteria

As a result of treatment using this protocol, the client may expect to be able to report:

1. Feeling less physical tension
2. Feeling more emotional control
3. Being more aware of his/her mood states and the ability to not overreact to them behaviorally
4. Being aware of how built up stress can trigger episodes of anxiety
5. Having a plan to reduce stress
6. Being able to use meditation and relaxation techniques independently

VI. Bibliography

Apóstolo, J. L. & Kolcaba, K. (2009). The effects of guided imagery on comfort, depression, anxiety, and stress of psychiatric inpatients with depressive disorders. *Psychiatric Nursing, 23*(6), 403-11.

Mullen, J. (Ed.) (2004). *Manual of Rating Scales for the Assessment of Mood Disorders*. Wilmington, DE: AstraZeneca Pharmaceuticals.

Beck, A. & Weishaar, M. (2005). Cognitive therapy. In R. J. Corsini and D. Wedding (Eds.), *Current Psychotherapies*, 238-268. Belmont, CA: Thomson Brooks/Cole Publishing.

Bennett, M. P., Rosenberg, L., Zeller, J., & McCann, J. (2003). The effect of mirthful laughter on stress and natural killer cell activity. *Alternative Therapies, 9*(2), 38-44.

Beyond Ordinary Nursing (2003). San Mateo, CA. www.integrativeimagery.com.

Bonadies, V. (2009). Guided imagery as a therapeutic recreation modality to reduce pain and anxiety. *Therapeutic Recreation Journal, 43*(2), 43-55.

burlingame, j., & Blaschko, T. M. (2010). *Assessment Tools for Recreational Therapy, 4th Ed.* Enumclaw, WA. Idyll Arbor, Inc.

Davis, M., Eshelman, R., & McKay, M. (2008). *The Relaxation and Stress Reduction Workbook.* Oakland, CA: New Harbinger Publications.

Dossey, B. (1995). Using imagery to help your patient heal. *American Journal of Nursing, 5*, 41-46.

Glaser, R. (2005). Stress-associated immune dysregulation and its importance for human health: A personal history of psychoneuroimmunology. *Brain, Behavior and Immunology, 19*(1), 3-11.

Grossman, P., Niemann, L., Schmidt, S., & Walach, H. (2004). Mindfulness-based stress reduction and health benefits: A meta-analysis. *Journal of Psychosomatic Research, 57*, 35-43.

Irwin, M., Patterson, T., Smith, T. L., Caldwell, C., Brown, S. A., & Gillin, J. C. (1990). Grant I: Reduction of immune function in life stress and depression. *Biological Psychiatry, 27*, 22-30.

King, J. V. (1988). A holistic technique to lower anxiety: Relaxation with guided imagery. *Journal of Holistic Nursing, 6*, 16-20.

Knight, C. (2006). Group for individuals with traumatic histories: Practice considerations for social workers. *Social Work, 51*(1), 20-30.

Manzoni, G., Pagnini, F., Castelnuovo, G., & Molinari, E. (2008). Relaxation training for anxiety: A ten-year systematic review with meta-analysis. *BMC Psychiatry, 8*(1), art. No. 41.

McCain, N. L., & Smith, J. C. (1994). Stress and coping in the context of psychoneuroimmunology: A holistic framework for nursing practice and research. *Archives of Psychiatric Nursing, 8*(4), 221-227.

Mullen, J., Endicott, J., Hirshfeld, R., Yonkers, K., Targum, S., & Bullinger, A. (2004). *Manual of Rating Scales for the Assessment of Mood Disorders.* Wilmington, DE: Astra Zeneca Pharmaceuticals LP.

Oei, T. P. S., & Brown, A. (2006). Components of group processes: Have they contributed to the outcome of mood and anxiety disorder patients in a group cognitive-behaviour therapy program? *American Journal of Psychotherapy, 60*(1), 53-70.

Porter, J. E. (2007). *The Thinking Person's Stress Management Workbook.* Audio Vision/Stress Stop.com. 2007.

Smith, J. C. (2005). *Relaxation, Meditation and Mindfulness: A Mental Health Practitioner's Guide to New and Traditional Approaches.* New York, NY: Springer.

Dementia of the Alzheimer's Type

I. Diagnosis

Dementia of the Alzheimer's Type

II. Assessment Criteria

Cognitive functioning is evaluated relative to memory impairment, orientation, and executive functioning (skills such as planning, initiation, organizing, sequencing, abstract thinking, and judgment). Clients' social and physical functioning is also evaluated including evaluation of past leisure interests. The agency's screening assessment may be followed by the use of the Mini-Mental State Exam, the Therapeutic Recreation Activity Assessment (TRAA), or the Ohio Functional Assessment Battery, as indicated. Often, the client with dementia will be unable to respond to questions accurately. Interviewing family members may provide more useful information.

III. Symptoms

Dementia of the Alzheimer's type is marked by the following symptoms:

1. The development of multiple cognitive deficits manifested by both memory impairment and one of the following: aphasia, apraxia, or agnosia
2. Disturbance in executive functioning, e.g., planning, organizing, sequencing, abstracting
3. Social and occupational impairment represented by a decline from a previous level of functioning
4. Gradual onset of symptoms
5. Continuing cognitive decline
6. The presence of audio or visual hallucinations

IV. Process Criteria

Clients are generally admitted to a geriatric behavioral health setting because of behavioral disturbances or for hallucinations. Often the client becomes agitated because of the presence of the psychotic symptoms or out of a lack of understanding what is happening to him/her. As the treating physician is adjusting medications to decrease these disruptive behaviors, the role of the recreational therapist is to provide structured modalities that improve the client's ability to focus in the present and to improve mood through pleasurable activities. Some of these activities evoke agreeable memories from the client's past. Others help the client engage in meaningful activities. The enthusiasm and skill of the therapist in encouraging the client is important. A review of the client's past and current leisure interests guides the therapist to those activities that are of value to the client.

The recreational therapist will develop an individualized treatment plan, considering all subjective and objective information, and provide treatment to the client from among the following modalities:

1. Exercise
2. Reminiscence
3. Validation

4. Sensory stimulation
5. Structured tasks such as sorting, crafts, cooking, gardening
6. Music
7. Socialization activities

V. Outcome Criteria

At the completion of treatment the client will be able to:

1. Reduce agitation and control energy level
2. Relate to past experiences and verbalize about these experiences
3. Decrease negative behavior
4. Improve effective speech
5. Be able to evoke memories related to the subject for review
6. Increase focus to task
7. Increase interaction with peers through relevant speech and movement

VI. Bibliography

American Psychiatric Association. (2000). *Diagnostic and Statistical Manual of Mental Disorders (Fourth Edition, Text Revision)*. Washington, DC.

Bates, J., Boote, J., & Beverly, C. (2004). Psychosocial interventions for people with a mild dementing illness: A systematic review. *Journal of Advanced Nursing, 45*(6), 644-658.

Best-Martini, E., Weeks, M. A., & Wirth, P. (2011). *Long Term Care for Activity Professionals, Social Services Professionals, and Recreational Therapists, Sixth Ed.* Ravensdale, WA: Idyll Arbor.

Birren, J. E. & Deutchman, D. E. (1991). *Guiding Autobiography Groups for Older Adults*. Baltimore: Johns Hopkins Press.

Bohlmeijer, E., Roemer, M., Cuijpers, P., & Smit, F. (2007). The effects of reminiscence on psychological well-being in older adults: A meta-analysis. *Aging & Mental Health, 11*(3), 291-300.

Beuttner, L. & Fitzsimmons, S. 2003. *Dementia Practice Guidelines for Recreational Therapy: Treatment of Disturbing Behaviors*. Alexandria, VA: American Therapeutic Recreation Association.

Caperchione, C. & Mummery, K. (2006). The utilization of group process strategies as an intervention for the promotion of health-related physical activity in older adults. *Activities, Adaptation & Aging, 30*(4), 29-45.

Feil, N. (1993). *Validation Therapy*. Cleveland: Edward Feil Productions.

Feil, N. (1993). *The Validation Breakthrough: Simple Techniques for Communicating with People with Alzheimer's-Type Dementia*. Baltimore: Health Professions Press.

Gallo, J. J., Reichel, W., & Andersen, L. (1988). *Handbook of Geriatric Assessment*. Rockville: Aspen Publications.

Hurley, O. (1988). *Safe Therapeutic Exercise for the Frail Elderly: An Introduction*. Albany: The Center for the Study of Aging.

Kane, R. & Kane, R. (1981). *Assessing the Elderly: A Practical Guide to Measurement*. Lexington: Lexington Books.

Kemp, B. (1990). *Geriatric Rehabilitation*. Boston: College-Hill Press.

Keogh-Hoss, M. A. (1994). *Therapeutic Recreation Activity Assessment.* Ravensdale, WA: Idyll Arbor, Inc.

Mobily, K. (2008). *Strength Training for Older Adults: Workshop Manual.* University of Iowa.

Moniz-Cook, E. (2006). Cognitive stimulation and dementia. *Aging & Mental Health, 10*(3), 207-210.

Parker, S. D. & Will, C. (1993). *Activities for the Elderly Volume 2: A Guide to Working with Residents with Significant Physical and Cognitive Disabilities.* Ravensdale, WA: Idyll Arbor, Inc.

Scogin, F. & Prohaska, M. (1993). *Aiding Older Adults with Memory Complaints.* Sarasota: Professional Resource Press.

Spector, A., Davies, S., Woods, B., & Orrell, M. (2000). Reality orientation for dementia: A systematic review of the evidence for its effectiveness. *Gerontologist, 40*(2), 206-212.

Tanaka, K., Yamada, Y., Kobayashi, Y., Sonohara, K., Machida, A., Nakai, R., Kozaki, K., & Toba, K. (2007). Improved cognitive function, mood and brain blood flow in single photon emission computed tomography following individual reminiscence therapy in an elderly patient with Alzheimer's disease. *Geriatric Gerontology International, 7*, 305-309.

Youssef, F. (1990). The impact of group reminiscence counseling on a depressed elderly population. *Nurse Practitioner, 15*(4), 34-38.

Zgola, J. M. (1987). *Doing Things: A Guide to Programming Activities for Persons with Alzheimer's Disease and Related Disorders.* Baltimore: Johns Hopkins Press.

Program Protocols

A program protocol is a description of the specific treatment group that will be offered to a client such as gardening or stress management. Within each program there will be several potential activities or modalities that may be used according to the needs of the clients. These may also be considered group descriptions, but the program protocol will be broader in scope.

The activities described in the protocol may be considered prescriptive. This happens when one activity builds on skills developed in the previous activity. Or, the activities may be suggestive and permit flexibility by the therapist in choosing the appropriate activity for the client group.

The outline of the program protocol has seven parts:

1. Treatment modality
2. Rationale
3. Referral criteria
4. Risk management issues
5. Structure criteria
6. Process criteria
7. Outcome criteria
8. Credentialing required by staff
9. Bibliography of supporting material

The first part is the name of the program protocol. It should be broad enough to include several different activities or steps that will be provided, according to the assessed needs of the client group.

The second part of the program protocol is the rationale, a statement about why this intervention is needed. From a review of literature the therapist will identify client needs that are addressed by this intervention. For example, low energy and fatigue are among the documented symptoms of depression that may be improved by participation in an exercise program. The rationale should also include efficacy-based evidence that the particular modality has been shown to improve functioning in the targeted area. One example may be the evidence that developing a social support system decreases mental illness symptoms and help-seeking behavior. To meet health care standards the therapist will need to be able to provide scientifically documented rationales for the interventions being used.

Part three of the program protocol outline is referrals. Not all clients will benefit from participation in the activities of a particular program protocol. For instance, not everyone needs to develop skills in personal hygiene. This part of the protocol provides guidance for both the recreational therapist and the rest of the treatment team as to who should be treated with this protocol.

The fourth part of the program protocol is risk management. In this part the therapist identifies any possible safety liabilities that the client or the facility may incur as a result of participation. Exposure to risk is managed by identifying the risk, structuring the activity to reduce risk, and outlining steps to be taken if a risk occurs.

The fifth part of the program protocol is structure criteria. Structure criteria refer to the mechanics of the group. It includes:

- How long each group activity will take
- How many clients can engage in this modality
- How often the group will meet
- The staffing ratio
- What room/space arrangements are needed
- What specific activities will be used within that program

The sixth part of the program protocol is process criteria. Process criteria refer to the actions that the therapist will take. These actions may include instruction, discussion, demonstration, observation, assistance, listening, leadership, discussion facilitation, and reinforcement. While the structure criteria define a time frame for an activity, the process criteria describe what the therapist will be doing during each segment of the time frame.

The seventh part of the program protocol is outcome criteria. Outcome criteria refer to what benefits the clients will achieve from participation in the protocol, what knowledge they will gain, or what behavioral changes they could expect. These outcomes are a direct result of the structure and process criteria.

The eighth part of the program protocol is the credentialing criteria for staff who implement the protocol. At a minimum the credential is the Certified Therapeutic Recreation Specialist (CTRS) from the National Council for Therapeutic Recreation Certification. Some states also require licensure as a recreational therapist. However, some protocols may require additional training or specialization in, for instance, fitness or cognitive therapy. These additional trainings would be required by the facility and based on the facility's policies and procedures. Since there is no official credential for a paraprofessional in therapeutic recreation, we assume that a paraprofessional conducting parts of a program protocol is working under the supervision of a CTRS.

The last part of the program protocol outline is the bibliography. This information will guide other employees and administrators of the facility to where the evidence-based research can be found. Administrators are concerned about "best practices" and evidence-based research, which increase the efficiency and effectiveness of the delivery.

The program protocols included in this book may serve as guides. These protocols may be cross-referenced to other populations. A therapist may review one protocol written for a specific population group and adapt it for use with another population of clients. For instance, the Therapeutic Art program written for the child/adolescent population may be suitable for adult and geriatric groups. There may be some variations made in the use of focus or materials, such as avoiding use of scissors because of limitations in manual abilities with the elderly.

The following pages have examples of program protocols. Since they are in no way inclusive of all possible program protocols, we encourage the therapist to use these as a starting point for his/her facility's own set of program protocols.

Sample Program Protocol

I. Treatment Modality

Write in the name of the group or individual program.

II. Rationale

Cite from the current version of the *Diagnostic and Statistical Book for Mental Disorder* (*DSM-IV-TR*) the symptomatology that this program is designed to treat. Use citations from available efficacy-based research to support the need for this program.

III. Referral Criteria

Identify what kinds of clients will participate in this program. Particular diagnostic groups may be cited, or clients may be chosen according to assessed needs and symptoms observed. State any contraindications that exist for participation in this group.

IV. Risk Management

Consider what extraordinary organizational risk may be incurred by the health care organization, as well as any unusual personal risks that could be incurred by clients in the program. Suggest ways of controlling the possible risks through careful assessment, observation, procedures, or taking immediate action in response to untoward events.

V. Structure Criteria

State the structure for conducting the groups, e.g., length of group, frequency. List the specific treatment modules that may be used in the program.

VI. Process Criteria

List what steps the therapist will take, including content of the program and facilitation interventions.

VII. Outcome Criteria

Identify what outcomes the clients may anticipate if they complete the process and content of the group.

VIII. Credentialing

Since professional preparation reduces risks in programs, list any special certifications, clinical privileges, or special training the therapist must have to conduct this program. These special credentials may be facility-specific requirements or recommendations.

IX. Bibliography

Record what bibliographical references were used to develop this protocol. Special emphasis is placed on efficacy-based research.

Child/Adolescent Program Protocols

The following protocols are most appropriate for child and adolescent populations.

Therapeutic Art Program

I. Treatment Modality

Therapeutic Art Program

II. Rationale

Communication is very important in all aspects of life. However, children often do not have the language skills necessary to explain their complex thoughts and feelings. Art is a natural mode of communication that children rarely resist and that offers them a way to express themselves in a manner that is less threatening than verbal means. For example, art allows children who have experienced trauma and loss the opportunity to externalize emotions and events too painful to speak out loud and is one of the only means of conveying the complexities of the painful experiences, repressed memories, or unspoken fears, anxieties, or guilt. Therapeutic art allows children to put a voice to their pain.

While the actual art may say a great deal about the child who creates it, what are more important are the therapeutic benefits that the process provides. For instance, children who have Attention Deficit/Hyperactivity Disorder or Oppositional Defiant Disorder often have a difficult time concentrating on basic activities, but therapeutic art can engage the mind and emotions more effectively. This specific type of client will be too busy and focused on positive activities to worry about negative consequences, the passage of time, intrusive thoughts, or other emotional disturbances. In addition, therapeutic art will allow for more discussion and processing to take place about the specific symptoms the client presents.

It is possible that art stimulates neurological processes that, in conjunction with specific questions and debriefing techniques, may be helpful in resolving stress reactions and reducing anxiety, intrusive thoughts, and other posttraumatic effects (Siegel, 1999).

III. Referrals

Any client may be referred to this program as long as his/her behavior is not disruptive to the group. Individuals who exhibit disruptive behavior may benefit from similar activities conducted in an individual session.

IV. Risk Management

Clients will be screened daily in regards to appropriateness for this program. Clients will not be included in sessions if they are displaying self-harming behaviors, excessive aggression, or disruptive behaviors in an attempt to keep the specific client and other group members safe.

In addition, clients' allergies will also be taken into consideration when planning therapeutic art activities.

Finally, an inventory of supplies will be taken before and after each session when utilizing scissors, pencil sharpeners, or other sharp objects.

V.   Structure Criteria

The therapeutic art program will be conducted weekly in a quiet space for 45 to 60 minutes, depending on the attending skills of the group. Group size may vary, but should be limited to no more than eight individuals so all participants have equal opportunities to contribute to group discussions.

VI.   Process Criteria

The recreational therapist will utilize a variety of therapeutic art activities to provide opportunities to express feelings and emotions, minimize anxiety or stress, and promote social interactions with peers. The therapist should be aware of the each client's abilities and limitations so activities are appropriately planned to address each client's specific needs.

At the beginning of each session the therapist will welcome participants and explain that the purpose of the group is to "simply try your best." It is also important to explain that group members should not criticize other's work or share other's thoughts and feelings outside of the group setting. The session will begin by introducing a specific topic to be explored such as feelings, goal setting, positive self-image, or family dynamics. Once the topic is discussed and understood, a specific type of media will be introduced such as clay, oil pastels, or paint. The participant will then be given the majority of the session to create a work of art related to the specific topic out of the media provided. The last ten to fifteen minutes should be utilized for the clients to share their work of art with the group, but only if they are willing to. It is important to enforce "share by choice" principles so clients do not feel pressured to talk about difficult topics in front of peers. However, the recreational therapist must be willing to discuss this with the participant one-on-one or ask a mental health professional to follow up with the client.

Specific activities that can be used include:

1. Family sculptures
2. Life size collages about oneself
3. Painting/drawing the way a musical selection makes the client feel
4. Creating a timeline of one's life through drawing or locating pictures from magazines
5. Drawing a map of how to accomplish personal goals
6. Creating a personal superhero out of recycled materials (identifying the specific powers s/he would have)
7. Creating masks to reflect one's personality

VII. Outcome Criteria

As a result of participation in this program, the participant will:

1. Be able to identify various feelings and emotions
2. Display more confidence in self
3. Report reduced anxiety or stress
4. Be able to demonstrate improved communication skills
5. Interact with peers appropriately

VIII. Credentialing

The Certified Therapeutic Recreation Specialist conducting this program will be trained and deemed competent to lead a therapeutic art program. Competencies are defined by the recreational therapy department based on agency policies and procedures. Such competencies may include, but are not limited to, demonstrating the proper use of art supplies and materials, a basic knowledge of art methods, and skillfulness at facilitating group discussions.

IX. Bibliography

Siegel, D. (1999). *The Developing Mind*. New York: Guilford Press.

Davis, J. & Gardner, H. (1993). The arts and early childhood education: A cognitive developmental portrait of the young child as artist. In B. Spodek (Ed.). *Handbook of Research in Early Childhood Education*. New York: Macmillan.

Makin, S. R. (2000). *Therapeutic Art Directives and Resources*. London, England: Jessica Kingsley Publishers.

Pet Assisted Therapy

I. Treatment Modality

Pet Assisted Therapy

II. Rationale

Pet assisted therapy is the use of animals to attain certain goals in a professional therapeutic environment. Almost any animal can be used in a pet assisted program, as long as it is a pleasant and sociable animal. The animals can be used as a peaceful escape or as a learning tool.

Often an animal can be useful when beginning interactions with a client who is withdrawn because the animal acts as a distraction, helps calm the client, but still creates opportunities for discussion. There is evidence that a situation can be deemed less threatening to a child if an animal is present. This change in the child's view of the environment can make a recreational therapist seem friendlier and easier to talk to, which will allow for a stronger bond to be formed.

Pet assisted therapy can also be helpful with clients who have emotional disorders such as Attention Deficit/Hyperactivity Disorder, Oppositional Defiant Disorder, Depression, or Anxiety Disorder. Research has found that children with emotional disorders become more readily involved with animals than with people or tasks. Children often find it easier to practice non-aggressive voice tones, appropriate eye contact, and proper techniques for sharing and playing with an animal because the animal will not argue or reject them. These techniques, learned with an animal, can then be generalized to other human interactions.

Pet assisted therapy is also helpful with clients who have Oppositional Defiant Disorder and Conduct Disorder. This specific type of client typically displays repetitive patterns of behavior that violate the basic rights of others. The pet assisted therapy program can be directed at refocusing the child's aggressive and dominating actions towards caring and gentle actions in a relationship free of rejection and full of unconditional positive regard. The child can form a secure attachment with another living being that will contribute to his/her basic sense of trust and eventually be transferred to human relationships.

Overall, most children have an innate fascination and curiosity towards animals, so children often find it much easier to empathize and relate to animals because their actions are much more simple and obvious than the complex behaviors a human exhibits. The pet assisted therapy program may decrease anxiety, improve social skills, increase the ability to trust, and teach responsibility all while in an environment free of rejection or criticism.

III. Referrals

Any client may be referred to this program as long as the client does not have an extensive history of animal abuse or his/her behavior is not disruptive to the group. Individuals who are not appropriate for the group may benefit from similar activities conducted in an individual session.

IV. Risk Management

Clients will be screened daily in regards to appropriateness for this program. Clients will not be included in sessions if they are displaying self-harming behaviors, excessive aggression, or disruptive behaviors in an attempt to keep the specific client, other group members, and the animal safe.

In addition, clients' allergies will be taken into consideration when planning pet assisted therapy activities.

V. Structure Criteria

The pet assisted therapy program will be conducted for 60 minutes, once a week in a quiet room with minimal distractions. The group size may vary, but should be kept small enough so that all participants have frequent opportunities for interacting with the pets. An ideal group size would be six to eight individuals.

VI. Process Criteria

The recreational therapist will utilize a variety of pet assisted therapy activities to provide opportunities to minimize anxiety or stress, promote social interactions with animals and peers, and demonstrate empathy and responsibility. The therapist should be aware of each client's abilities and limitations so activities are appropriately planned to address each client's specific needs.

At the beginning of each session the therapist will welcome participants and explain that the purpose of the group is to "simply have fun." It is also important to explain appropriate handling techniques for the specific type of animal that is being utilized. Once the expectations are explained, the clients are given the remainder of the session to interact with the pet or pets. Conversations will be directed to the individuals' interests and related to typical interactions with humans.

Specific topics that can be discussed include:

1. Body language
2. Communication
3. Needs of animals
4. Hygiene
5. Relationships
6. Specific roles in a group

Some of the activities you could involve clients in include observing animal behavior, grooming pets, cleaning cages, feeding pets, and engaging pets in exercise.

VII. Outcome Criteria

As a result of participation in this program, the client will:

1. Report having fun
2. Be able to engage with various pets and explain how this relates to relationships with human beings in regards to communication, body language, and group roles
3. Demonstrate more calmness in the presence of an animal

VIII. Credentialing

The Certified Therapeutic Recreation Specialist will be deemed competent to lead a pet therapy program. Competencies are defined by the Recreational Therapy Department based on agency policies and procedures. Competencies may include, but are not limited to, demonstrating the proper care and handling techniques of the animals being utilized. Animals should be registered pet therapy animals through Therapy Dogs International (TDI), Delta Society (registers dogs and animals other than dogs), or another similar agency.

IX. Bibliography

Abdill, M. & Juppé, D. (2005). *Pets in Therapy: Animal Assisted Activities in Health Care Facilities.* Ravensdale, WA: Idyll Arbor.

Brooks, S. (2006). Animal-assisted psychotherapy and equine-assisted psychotherapy. In N. Webb (Ed.) *Working with Traumatized Youth in Child Welfare.* New York: Guildford Press.

Fine, A. H., Editor. (2010). *Handbook on Animal Assisted Therapy: Theoretical Foundations and Guidelines*, 3rd Edition. London, England: Academic Press/Elsevier.

Circus Performance Program

I. Treatment Modality

Circus Performance Program

II. Rationale

The circus performance program is a unique and active modality utilizing a variety of skills seen in the circus. Even though it appears this type of program is about learning new skills, what the individual learns about himself/herself along the way is much more important. This type of program is ideal for clients who exhibit attention difficulties, inability to express themselves, difficulty forming successful relationships, lack of self-esteem, and oppositional defiant behaviors. In this non-competitive environment, clients have the opportunity to set individual goals, solve problems, learn and practice various roles within a group, express feelings, make decisions, and reduce anxiety or stress.

Children with Attention Deficit/Hyperactivity Disorder often become bored easily and have a difficult time focusing on one task for any given period of time. Through the circus performance program the participants will have specific tasks they need to work on, but, if they get bored, they can move on to the next area of interest. Various tasks can be revisited as many times as the session allows. In addition, most of the circus tasks are very active and require a great deal of energy. This allows the individual a positive way to release the extra energy that often builds up.

The circus performance program is also ideal for clients that display oppositional defiant behaviors. These particular clients struggle to follow instruction from authority figures, blame others for their mistakes, and become angry easily. However, in this type of setting minimal instruction is given, the participants decide for themselves what activity they are going to engage in, and, if they become frustrated, they can move on to a different skill. The structure of these sessions is ideal for clients who present with oppositional defiant behaviors.

Circus skills appear to be an unusual concept, however, the benefits are endless and the program is easily adapted to fit the group.

III. Referrals

Any client may be referred to this program as long as his/her behavior is not disruptive to the group. Individuals who are disruptive may benefit from similar activities conducted in an individual session.

IV. Risk Management

Professional circus instructors should be utilized to assist with facilitation of these sessions due to the knowledge required to teach these skills safely.

Due to the physical and active nature of this program each individual's physical fitness level should be taken into consideration. Appropriate protective gear should be worn when utilizing stilts, rolling globe, or the tight rope. In addition, individuals' allergies should be taken into consideration, especially when working with balloons.

V. Structure Criteria

The circus performance program will be conducted for 60 minutes, once a week in a large room free of distractions. The group size may vary, but should be small enough so that all participants have frequent opportunities to try out the props being utilized. An ideal group size should be no more than 10 participants.

VI. Process Criteria

Prior to beginning circus performance groups, a professional circus instructor should be identified to work with the recreational therapist and assist in planning each session based on the specific needs of the clients being served.

The professional circus instructor will utilize a variety of circus skills to provide opportunities to set individual goals, solve problems, learn and practice various roles within a group, express feelings, make decisions, and reduce anxiety or stress. The recreational therapist acts as support to the professional circus instructor by directing discussions and offering assistance to the instructor and participants.

At the beginning of each session the recreational therapist will welcome participants and explain that the purpose of the group is to "simply try your best." It is also important to explain that group members should not criticize other's ability, but instead help each other out and utilize encouraging words.

The session starts with three circle activities: a general question, stretching, and a team-building exercise. The purpose of the general question is to allow the group members to get to know each other better and find things they have in common with one another. Some sample questions include: share one thing you learned today, what is your favorite food, what are you good at, or what is your favorite animal. The participants are then engaged in basic stretching exercises to warm up their muscles for the remainder of the activities. The group then moves on to a team-building exercise. This is important because it helps the group bond, increases the energy level of the group, and sets the tone for the remainder of the session. Some sample activities that can be utilized include group juggling, name and gesture, or pass the squeeze. These activities are typically fairly quick, but really give the group a sense of accomplishment.

Finally, the professional circus instructor introduces the new skill to the group and the participants are given the remainder of the session to work on this particular skill and any others that have been introduced in previous sessions. The last ten to fifteen minutes should be utilized for the clients to share their perspective on this group experience. Some important leading questions the recreational therapist should ask include: what did you do really well today, what were your struggles today, or what are your personal goals for next week. It is important to enforce "share by choice" principles so clients do not feel pressured to talk about difficult topics in front of peers. However, the recreational therapist must be willing to discuss this with the client one-on-one or ask a mental health professional to follow up with the client.

Specific activities that can be used include:

1. Balancing feathers
2. Juggling scarves/balls/clubs
3. Spinning plates
4. Making balloon animals

5. Roll-a-bolla boards
6. Rolling globes
7. Stilts
8. Tight rope
9. Clowning

VII. Outcome Criteria

The client will:

1. Increase self-esteem
2. Demonstrate appropriate social skills
3. Identify a variety of coping skills
4. Manage frustration or anger
5. Identify something s/he has achieved

VIII. Credentialing

A professional circus instructor should be utilized to assist with the facilitation of this program due to the knowledge required to teach these skills safely. A Certified Therapeutic Recreation Specialist assisting with the circus performance group should be deemed competent to facilitate these sessions. Competencies are defined by the recreational therapy department based on the agency policies and procedures. Competencies may include, but are not limited to, a general knowledge of the skills being taught to the clients and an awareness of important safety guidelines. The CTRS will be physically fit to be able to assist.

IX. Bibliography

American Psychiatric Association. (2000). *Diagnostic and Statistical Manual of Mental Disorders*
        (Fourth Edition, Text Revision). Washington, DC.
Social circus: A guide to good practices.
        http://sosiaalinensirkus.fi/english/uploads/images/social_circus_handbook_2011.pdf. Retrieved:
        1-19-12.

Community Integration

I. Treatment Modality

Community Integration

II. Rationale

The diagnosis of mental illness comes with the additional burden of a negative label. Research suggests that the community reacts disapprovingly toward those diagnosed with mental illness. In turn, these stigmas affect an individual's self-esteem, ability to form relationships, social acceptance, and even job opportunities.

Community integration is a modality utilized to assist a child with mental illness or behavioral issues in normalizing his/her behavior in public settings. This is accomplished by engaging the client in positive community leisure choices, while practicing appropriate and acceptable social etiquette. In turn, this leads to an increase in self-esteem, positive views of the self, increased ability to form relationships, and social acceptance.

In addition, it is extremely important to provide a wide variety of community integration sessions so the child understands appropriate social behaviors in all settings. For example, when attending a baseball game it is completely acceptable to wear a team t-shirt, jeans, and cheer loudly when your team scores. However, when attending a play you may want to wear nice khakis, a polo, and remain quiet until it is time to applaud.

III. Referrals

Since this community integration is taking place in a public setting, additional considerations need to be taken into account when clients are referred to this program. Clients must be able to interact appropriately in a group setting, understand appropriate social etiquette, and have identified coping skills to utilize when upset or frustrated. If a client has not yet accomplished these tasks, s/he should not be included in this program to ensure his/her safety, as well as that of the other group and community members.

IV. Risk Management

The recreational therapist will ensure that all participants are screened for the intervention. Individuals will not be included in sessions if they are displaying self-harming behaviors, excessive aggression, or disruptive behaviors. This is required to keep that individual, other group members, and community members safe.

Because of the risk of elopement, additional staff will be on hand to assist with supervision and teaching moments.

Specific allergies and medical conditions will be taken into consideration when planning the community integration sessions.

V. Structure Criteria

The community integration program will be conducted at least once a week. The time and location will be determined based on the interests of the group members involved. Additional staff should be on hand to assist with supervision and teaching moments.

VI. Process Criteria

The recreational therapist utilizes a variety of community outings to assist in improving self-esteem and appropriate social behaviors and to foster the formation of appropriate relationships.

At the beginning of each session, the therapist will welcome participants and educate them on expectations and appropriate social etiquette for the particular community setting. The recreational therapist will also explain that the purpose of this session is to have fun and possibly add a new leisure activity to the participants' interests. The group will then depart for the community outing.

It is important to process the activity afterwards to identify the areas the participants struggled with and different ways to overcome these obstacles. It is also important to praise an individual for any difficult situations that s/he was able to work through while on this outing.

The activities that can be utilized for the community integration program are dependent on the interests of the group. However, some examples of outings include:

1. Sporting events
2. Going out to eat
3. Visiting a library
4. Going to a movie
5. Roller skating

The recreational therapist could also arrange guest speakers or shows to visit the facility if the group is not advanced enough to go off grounds.

VII. Outcome Criteria

The individual will:

1. Demonstrate improved socials skills
2. Increase self-esteem
3. Develop appropriate relationships
4. Report having "fun"

VIII. Credentialing

The Certified Therapeutic Recreation Specialist will be deemed competent, as defined by the recreational therapy department and in accordance with the policies and procedures of the agency. Competencies may include, but are not limited to, a knowledge of the location where the event will take place and proper etiquette in such a place. Additional staff and/or volunteers will also be included to assist with supervision and teaching moments.

IX. Bibliography

Disability rights education & defense fund. http://www.dredf.org/international/paper_r-k.html. Retrieved 12-12-11.

Stigma of mental illness. http://www.sma.org.sg/smj/4203/4203a4.pdf. Retrieved 12-15-11.

Normalizing as the opposite of labeling. http://www.soc.ucsb.edu/faculty/scheff/77.pdf. Retrieved 12-15-11.

Adult Program Protocols

The following protocols are most appropriate for adult populations.

Fitness Program
(Contributed by Marcia Smith)

I.   Treatment Modality

Fitness Program

II.   Rationale

Studies have shown that light to moderate exercise can combat many common health issues such as high blood pressure, weight gain, high cholesterol, and diabetes. The American College of Sport Medicine and the American Heart Association (2012), recommend that adults under 65 years of age engage in:

- moderately intense cardiovascular exercise 150 minutes a week (30 minutes a day, five days a week)

or

- vigorously intense cardiovascular exercise 75 minutes a week

Moderate intensity is defined as working hard enough to raise your heart rate and break a sweat, yet still being able to carry on a conversation. It should be noted that to lose weight or maintain weight loss, 60 to 90 minutes of physical activity may be necessary. Also recommended as part of the exercise are eight to ten strength-training exercises, eight to twelve repetitions of each exercise, twice a week.

Many individuals with mental illnesses have a sedentary lifestyle which contributes to health conditions. They may also experience many symptoms secondary to their primary psychiatric diagnoses. Symptoms often reduced and managed with light to moderate exercise include fatigue, poor sleep, difficulty concentrating, depression, and anxiety. Engaging in exercise can also provide a distraction from negative and positive symptoms associated with schizophrenia. Exercising consistently has been proven to enhance the overall quality of life.

III. Referrals

Clients referred to an exercise program, per the agency's policy, may exhibit the following symptoms:

1. Fatigue
2. Depression
3. Anxiety
4. Difficulty concentrating
5. Poor sleep
6. Weight gain
7. Medically diagnosed high blood pressure, high cholesterol, diabetes, or decreased bone density

IV. Risk Management

Once a medical clearance to exercise is obtained, the client may attend the group. However, the therapist leading the group should evaluate the clients on the day of the group to determine their ability to safely participate that day. The therapist should check for clients who are, for example, experiencing any pain or discomfort or are light headed or dizzy. The therapist should determine that clients are wearing proper footwear and clothing, and that drinking water is easily available. Finally, the therapist should monitor the use of equipment for safety to minimize the risk of injury during the exercise group.

Because of the effect some medications can have on heart rate and blood pressure, traditional ways of monitoring heart rate and blood pressure may not be useful. Therapists therefore need to be aware of other methods for evaluating exertion such as the Borg Perceived Rate of Exertion. This scale ranging from 6 (very light) to 20 (extremely hard) is used to evaluate level of exertion during exercise.

Any equipment used should have regular maintenance and be evaluated as safe to use. The room should be clean, well lit, and free of obstacles. All equipment should be cleaned (wiped down) after each use, using an antiseptic solution. The therapist should observe clients to assure that the exercises and techniques are being completed safely. Any incidents that occur during the group should be reported and documented per agency policies and procedures.

V. Structure Criteria

The exercise group is conducted for one hour a minimum of three days per week in the fitness center/recreation area.

A complete fitness program incorporates endurance, strength, and flexibility. Endurance occurs when using the large muscle groups during prolonged and rhythmic aerobic activity such as walking and running. Strength training involves weightlifting and/or resistance exercises. Flexibility (stretching) is important for range of motion and is an essential health component. Because clients with mental illnesses tend to be sedentary, it is important to design an exercise program that addresses the needs of individuals considered "de-conditioned" and not provide exercises that raise the heart rate above 40%-60% of their target heart rate.

The exercise group should include the following:

1. Warm up (at least five minutes)
2. Cardiovascular activity (at least 20-30 minutes)
3. Strength training (at least twice per week targeting the main muscle groups)
4. Cool down — at least five minutes and should include light stretching (The cool down is critical to lowering the heart rate and to avoid pooling of blood in the legs. Following exercise the client should **not** be allowed to immediately sit but should walk for up to five minutes before sitting.)
5. Time for discussion or demonstration of exercises, reviewing hand-out materials

VI. Process Criteria

The therapist will:

1. Assess each client for participation prior to the group
2. Make sure the space used is free of hazards
3. Ensure that equipment is clean and in safe operational condition
4. Teach the benefits of exercise for overall health and managing symptoms

5. Develop and conduct a program that includes a warm up, cardiovascular exercise, strength training, and a cool down
6. Teach clients how to calculate maximum heart rate
7. Teach clients how to take their pulse (heart rate)
8. Discuss community resources
9. Provide written materials as needed

VII. Outcome Criteria

The client will:

1. Verbalize an understanding of the benefits of exercise on overall health and well being
2. Identify the method of exercise s/he finds most enjoyable
3. Identify how exercise has decreased symptoms
4. Verbalize those exercises that help manage symptoms and improve health
5. Demonstrate correct exercise techniques
6. Demonstrate the ability to take heart rate
7. Demonstrate an understanding of the impact of medications on heart rate and blood pressure during exercise
8. Verbalize how to maintain an exercise program following discharge

VIII. Credentialing

Certified Therapeutic Recreation Specialists conducting fitness programs should be trained and deemed competent to lead an exercise group. Competencies are defined by the recreational therapy department based on the agency policies and procedures. Competencies may include, but are not limited to, demonstrating the proper use of any exercise equipment available, basic knowledge of exercise principles and methods, calculating maximum heart rate, and taking a pulse.

IX. Bibliography

American College of Sport Medicine. (2008). *ACSM Guidelines for Exercise Testing and Prescription, 8th ed.* Philadelphia, PA: Lippincott Williams & Wilkins.

American College of Sport Medicine. (2010). *Resource Manual for Guidelines for Exercise Testing and Prescription, 6th ed.* Philadelphia, PA: Lippincott Williams & Wilkins.

American Heart Association. (2012). American Heart Association guidelines for physical activity. http://www.heart.org/HEARTORG/GettingHealthy/PhysicalActivity/StartWalking/American-Heart-Association-Guidelines_UCM_307976_Article.jsp. Retrieved August 25, 2012.

Dustman, R. E., Ruhling, R. O., Russell, E. M., Shearer, D. E., Bonekat, H. W., Shigeoka, J. W., et al. (1984). Aerobic exercise training and improved neuropsychological function of older individuals. *Neurobiology of Aging, 5,* 35-42.

Howley, E. T., & Franks, B. (1992). *Health Fitness Instructor's Handbook, 2nd ed.* Champaign, IL Human Kinetics.

U.S. Department of Health and Human Services (January 2010). *The Surgeon General's Vision for a Healthy and Fit Nation.* Rockville, MD: U.S. Department of Health and Human Services, Office of the Surgeon General.

American College of Sport Medicine (ACSM). www.acsm.org.

American Council on Exercise.www.acefitness.org.

National Strength Professionals Association (NSPA). www.nspainc.com.

National Strength & Conditioning Association. www.nsca-lift.org.

Leisure Education Program

I.   Treatment Modality

Leisure Education Program

II.   Rationale

Improvement of perceived well being through participation in a leisure education program has been suggested by Skalko (1982). Significant improvement of perceived leisure competence with the use of a leisure education program was identified by Searle and Mohna (1993). Bullock and Howe (1991) found improvement in behavioral functioning, adjustment to disability, autonomy, and quality of life after clients participated in a reintegration program utilizing leisure education. The meaning that we find through leisure activities can be helpful when healing from traumatic events (Park & Folkman, 1997).

III.   Referrals

Clients are referred to this program who have been identified, through a comprehensive assessment, as having limitations or deficits in one or more of the following areas:

1.   Leisure awareness
2.   Leisure attitude
3.   Leisure skills
4.   Social appropriateness
5.   Group interaction skills
6.   Sub-optimal recreation participation patterns

Clients who are not directable because of severe psychosis or intrusive behaviors are contraindicated.

IV.   Risk Management

When gross motor activities are used in these programs, clients will be assessed beforehand for any possible contraindications. Otherwise, there are no presumed risks.

V.   Structure Criteria

The leisure education program will be conducted for 60 minutes daily in the group treatment room. Modules will address and further assess the following areas:

1.   Leisure awareness
2.   Leisure attitude
3.   Leisure skills
4.   Social appropriateness
5.   Group interaction skills
6.   Recreation participation
7.   Recreation resources

VI. Process Criteria

In some settings, such as outpatient behavioral health models, there is more time to accomplish all of the process criteria identified below. This is more challenging in the short-term setting. It may be helpful to group the clients into smaller groups, based on assessed needs, or to identify one or two criteria on which the group can effectively focus in a reasonable amount of time.

The recreational therapist will assure that all clients are medically screened for the intervention and that the space is free of potential hazards. Paper and pencil exercises, role playing, leisure games, skill teaching, or group discussion may be among the techniques used.

The recreational therapist will:

1. Assist the client in identifying his/her knowledge of leisure appropriate to future leisure needs
2. Assist the client in identifying his/her behaviors and/or feelings toward leisure involvement
3. Assist the client in identifying his/her leisure skills and the potential for the acquisition of additional skills
4. Assist the client in identifying specific social behaviors which affect his/her ability to function effectively in leisure activities
5. Assist the client in acquiring interaction skills to participate in various types of individual and/or group situations
6. Assist the client in active participation in recreational activities
7. Assist the client in identifying personal and community resources for use after discharge

VII. Outcome Criteria

The client will:

1. Identify personal benefits of leisure involvement
2. List leisure strengths and weaknesses
3. Establish expectations and goals regarding leisure involvement
4. Identify his/her disposition toward leisure and recreation and at least two additional ways to direct future involvement
5. Inventory present leisure skills and express willingness to develop new ones
6. Display self-directed, socially acceptable behaviors in regards to manners, personal hygiene and dress, courteousness, and tolerance for others
7. Interact cooperatively and competitively in socially acceptable ways
8. Participate actively for the duration of the program without direct prompting from staff
9. Develop a plan to utilize personal and community resources after discharge

VIII. Credentialing

The therapist will hold national certification as a Certified Therapeutic Recreation Specialist from the National Council for Therapeutic Recreation Certification.

IX. Bibliography

Bullock, C. C. & Howe, C. Z. (1991). A model therapeutic recreation program for the reintegration of persons with disabilities in the community. *Therapeutic Recreation Journal, 25*(1) 7-17.

Coyle, C. P., Kinney, W. B., Riley, R., & Shank, J. (eds.) (1991). *Benefits of Therapeutic Recreation: A Consensus View.* Ravensdale, WA: Idyll Arbor, Inc.

Iwasaki, Y., Coyle, C., Shank, J., Salzer, M., Baron, D., Messina, E., Mitchell, L., Ryan, A., Koons, G., & Kishbauch, G. (2010). Exploring the role of leisure in recovery from mental illness. Abstracts from the 2010 American Therapeutic Recreation Association Research Institute. Hattiesburg, LA: ATRA.

Kloseck, M. & Crilly, R. (1997). *Leisure Competence Measure.* London, Ontario: Leisure Competence Measure Data System.

Park. C. L. & Folkman, S. (1997). Meaning in the context of stress and coping. *Review of General Psychology, 1*(2), 115-144.

Searle, M. S. & Mahon, M. J. (1993). The effects of a leisure education program on selected social-psychological variables: A three months follow-up investigation. *Therapeutic Recreation Journal*, 27 (1), 9-21.

Skalko, T. K. (1982). The effects of leisure education programs on the perceived leisure well-being of psychiatrically impaired active army personnel. Unpublished doctoral dissertation. University of Maryland: College Park, MD.

Friendship Development

I. Treatment Modality

Friendship Development

II. Rationale

Clients with depressive disorders, thought disorders, and personality disorders are at high risk for friendship disorders because inappropriate social behaviors are often part of the symptomatology of mental illness. Turner (1981) and Leavy (1983) found an association between the absence of social supports and increased psychological stress. In an extensive review of the literature, Antonucci (1989) found evidence that a social support system is related to a variety of cost-effective outcomes, including a decrease in mental illness symptoms, a reduction in help-seeking behavior, and a reduced need for hospitalization and shorter lengths of stay when admitted. Lehman and Steinwachs (2003) and Mojtabai, Nicholson, and Carpenter (1998) have reported that cognitive behavioral therapy has been shown to be an effective tool in psychosocial rehabilitation. Recent studies have shown a lower risk of developing dementia among people who have more social support (Fratiglioni et al, 2000), (Holtzman et al, 2004), (Seeman et al, 2001), and (Zunzunegui et al, 2003).

III. Referrals

Clients will be referred to the friendship development program who:

1. Have difficulty initiating and sustaining social conversations
2. Hold dysfunctional beliefs about the nature of friends and friendships
3. Report a narrow field of social supports

Clients who are non-directable because of severe psychotic symptoms or intrusive behaviors are contraindicated for this program.

It is presumed that clients have been introduced to the cognitive therapy process and have learned to use the daily mood log in other treatment groups.

IV. Risk Management

This program does not present organizational risk or risks to clients.

V. Structure Criteria

The friendship development program will meet daily for sixty-minute sessions. Three modules comprise the program:

1. Modifying dysfunctional beliefs
2. Improving social skills
3. Developing a social support system

VI. Process Criteria

For Session One the recreational therapist will:

1. Ask clients to identify thoughts they hold about the nature of friendship or about themselves or others in a friendship
2. Assist clients in the use of the daily mood log to restructure dysfunctional beliefs
3. Assign homework

For Session Two the recreational therapist will:

1. Distribute literature and lead discussion about non-verbal communication, how to start a conversation, and the importance of giving and receiving feedback
2. Assign role playing situations, process results with group
3. Assign homework

For Session Three the recreational therapist will:

1. Ask clients to identify lapsed social supports from the past that they can re-establish
2. Ask clients to identify appropriate and safe places and resources where they can make friends
3. Use problem-solving techniques with clients to overcome external barriers to achieving friends (e.g., transportation)
4. Assign homework

VII. Outcome Criteria

The client will:

1. Relate functional beliefs about the nature of friends and friendships
2. Exhibit improved ability to initiate conversations, give and receive feedback, and understand nonverbal communication cues
3. Identify a plan to seek social supports in the community

VIII. Credentialing

Therapists must demonstrate knowledge and skill in the use of cognitive therapy techniques and will be credentialed as a Certified Therapeutic Recreation Specialist by the National Council for Therapeutic Recreation Certification.

IX. Bibliography

Antonucci, T. C. (1989). Social support influences on the disease process. In L. Carstensen and J. Neale (Eds.). *Mechanisms of Psychological Influence on Physical Health.* 23-41. New York: Plenum Press.

Bellack, A. S. (2004). Skills training for people with severe mental illness. *Psychiatric Rehabilitation Journal, 27*(4), 375-391.

Bellack, A. S., Mueser, K. T., Gingerich, S., & Agresta, J. (2004). *Social Skills Training for Schizophrenia: A Step-by-Step Guide* (2nd ed.). New York: Guilford Press.

Bond, G. R. & Campbell, K. (2008). Evidence-based practices for individuals with severe mental illness. *Journal of Rehabilitation, 74*(2), 33-44.

Burns, D. D. (1989). *The Feeling Good Handbook.* New York: Wm. Morrow & Company, Inc.

Fratiglioni, L., Wang, H., Ericsson, K., Maytan, M., & Winblad, B. (2000). Influence of social network on occurrence of dementia: A community-based longitudinal study. *The Lancet, 355*, 1315-1319.

Gabor, D. (1983). *How to Start a Conversation and Make Friends*. New York: Simon and Schuster.

Holtzman, R. E., Rebok, G. W., Saczynski, J. S., Kouzis, A. C., Wilcox Doyle, K., & Eaton, W. W. (2004). Social network characteristics and cognition in middle-aged and older adults. *The Journals of Gerontology. Series B, Psychological Sciences and Social Sciences*, 59, 278-284.

Kurtz, M. M. & Mueser, K. T. (2008). A meta-analysis of controlled research on social skills training for schizophrenia. *Journal of Consulting and Clinical Psychology*, 76(30), 491-504.

Leavy, R. L. (1983). Social support and psychological disorder. *Journal of Community Psychology, 11*, 3-21.

Lehman, A. F. & Steinwachs, D. M. (2003). Evidence-based psychological practices in schizophrenia: Lessons from the patient outcomes research team (PORT) project. *Journal of the American Academy of Psychoanalysis and Dynamic Psychiatry, 31*, 141-154.

Mueller, D. R. & Bellack, A. S. (2007). Social skills training in recreational rehabilitation of schizophrenia patients. *American Journal of Recreation Therapy, 4*(5), 11-19.

Mojtabai, R., Nicholson, R. A., & Carpenter, B. N. (1998). Role of psychosocial treatment in management of schizophrenia: A meta-analytic review of controlled outcome studies. *Schizophrenia Bulletin, 24,* 569-587.

Seeman, T. E., Lusignolo, T. M., Albert, M., & Berkman, L. (2001). Social relationships, social support, and patterns of cognitive aging in healthy, high-functioning older adults: MacArthur studies of successful aging. *Health Psychology*, 20, 243-255.

Turner, R. J. (1981). Social support as a contingency in psychological well-being. *Journal of Health and Social Behavior, 22*, 357-367.

Young, J. T. (1986). A cognitive-behavioral approach to friendship disorders. In V. J. Derlego & B. A. Winstead. *Friendship in Social Interaction*, 247-276. New York: Springer-Verlag.

Zimbardo, P. (1977). *Shyness: What It Is. What to Do About It.* Reading, MA: Wesley Publishing Company.

Zunzunegui, M. V., Alvarado, B. E., Del Ser, T., & Otero, A. (2003). Social networks, social integration, and social engagement determine cognitive decline in community-dwelling Spanish older adults. *The Journals of Gerontology, 58,* S93-S10.

Stress Management and Relaxation

I. Treatment Modality

Stress Management and Relaxation

II. Rationale

While there are complex psychobiological causes of mental illness, it can be argued that cumulative stress or significant stressful events can precipitate or aggravate acute episodes of illness. According to the American Institute of Stress, up to 90% of all medical appointments are related to how we handle stress in our lives.

Matheny et al (1986) found social skills training, problem-solving, cognitive restructuring, and relaxation training to be among the more effective treatments for stress-related disorders. They suggest a treatment program that includes stress monitoring, marshaling resources (assertiveness training, confronting and dealing with issues), cognitive therapies, and tension reduction (relaxation and meditation training, exercise).

In a clinical trial, Herbert Benson et al (1980) compared subjects using three different modalities — medication, meditation, and progressive muscle relaxation. After five months, they found the meditation group showed significantly more symptom reduction than other groups. In addition, subjects showed improvement on the symptom checklist SCL-90-R in every one of the symptom scales, including somatization, depression, anxiety, hostility ($p < 0.001$ each), interpersonal sensitivity, paranoid ideation, psychoticism ($p < 0.01$ each), and obsessive-compulsive and phobic anxiety ($p < 0.05$ each).

III. Referrals

Clients will be referred to this program if they have depressive disorders with or without personality disorders and/or report significant stresses in their lives.

It is helpful if clients have been introduced to the cognitive therapy process and cognitive distortions.

IV. Risk Management

Clients who are not indicated for this program include those with organic mental disturbances or acute episodes of psychosis. Several categories of clients deserve special consideration. Clients who have dissociative disorders may require medical authorization before beginning any meditation or relaxation techniques. Those who have been sexually abused may feel more vulnerable during relaxation and meditation activities. They may want to self-select out of this part of the program or engage in such activities apart from the group. Finally, clients who have active seizure disorders should have medical approval before starting relaxation/meditation.

V. Structure Criteria

The Stress Management and Relaxation program will meet three days a week for 60 minutes each day. There will be three modules, each including a 40-minute psychoeducational component and a 20-minute experiential tension reduction session. Modules will include:

1. Stress monitoring, followed by progressive muscle relaxation

2. Developing stress management resources, followed by mindfulness meditation
3. Cognitive restructuring, followed by a guided imagery exercise

VI. Process Criteria

The recreational therapist will assure that all clients are medically screened for the intervention and that the space is free of potential hazards.

The recreational therapist will:

1. Assist clients in identifying sources of stress and biopsychosocial symptoms of stress
2. Lead clients in progressive muscle relaxation
3. Assist the group in identifying helpful strategies for managing stress, including but not limited to: developing support systems, time management, use of play, setting priorities, being assertive (The therapist may refer clients to community resources or literature where they may learn more about these strategies.)
4. Instruct clients in mindfulness meditation
5. Lead discussion of cognitive responses to stress and appropriate rational responses
6. Instruct clients in a guided imagery exercise

VII. Outcome Criteria

The client will:

1. Be able to identify symptoms for self-monitoring of stress
2. Be able to perform progressive muscle relaxation
3. Be able to identify effective coping strategies for self-management and list appropriate resources for additional help after discharge
4. Be able to independently perform mindfulness meditation
5. State a rational response to thoughts about stress
6. Be able to independently perform guided imagery

VIII. Credentialing

The Certified Therapeutic Recreation Specialist will have demonstrated training and competence in stress management theory and relaxation training, as well as a thorough knowledge of cognitive behavioral therapy.

IX. Bibliography

Baldwin, B. (1985). *It's All In Your Head: Lifestyle Management Strategies for Busy People.* Wilmington, NC: Direction Dynamics.

Benson, H. (1975). *Relaxation Response.* New York. Avon Books.

Benson, H. & Stuart, E. (1992). *The Wellness Book: A Comprehensive Guide to Maintaining Health and Treating Stress Related Illness.* New York: Birch Lane Press.

Benson, H., Kutz, I., & Borysenko, J. (1985). Meditation and psychotherapy: A rationale for the integration of dynamic psychotherapy, the relaxation response, and mindfulness meditation. *American Journal of Psychiatry, 142*(1) 1-8.

Carrigan, P. G., Collinger, H. Jr., Benson, H., Robinson, H., Wood, L.W., Lehrer, P. M., Woolfolf, R. L., & Cole, J. W. (1980). The use of meditation-relaxation techniques for the management of stress in a working population. *Journal of Occupational Medicine, 22*(4), 221-231.

Coyle, C. P., Kinney, W. B., Riley, R., Shank, J. (Eds.) (1991). *Benefits of Therapeutic Recreation: A Consensus View.* Ravensdale, WA: Idyll Arbor, Inc.

DeVries, H. A. (1987). Tension reduction with exercise. In Wm. P. Morgan and S. E. Goldston (eds.) *Exercise and Mental Health.* Washington, DC: Hemisphere Publishing.

Glaser, R. (2005). Stress-associated immune dysregulation and its importance for human health: A personal history of psychoneuroimmunology. *Brain, Behavior and Immunology, 19*(1): 3-11.

Karp, J. E., Shega, J. W., Morone, N. E., & Weiner, D. K. (2008). Advances in understanding the mechanisms and management of persistent pain in older adults. *British Journal of Anesthesia, 101*(1), 111-120.

Matheny, K. S., Aycock, D. W., Pugh, J., Curlette, W. L., & Silva Cannella, K. A. (1986). Stress coping: A qualitative and quantitative synthesis and implications for treatment. *The Counseling Psychologist, 14*(4) 499-549.

McCain, N. L. & Smith, J. C. (1994). Stress and coping in the context of psychoneuroimmunology: A holistic framework for nursing practice and research. *Archives of Psychiatric Nursing, 8*(4), 221-227.

Robins, J. L., McCain, N. L., Gray, D. P., Elswick, R. K. Jr., Walter, J. M., & McDade, E. (2006). Research on psychoneuroimmunology: Tai Chi as a stress management approach for individuals with HIV disease. *Applied Nursing Research, 19*(1), 2-9.

Stephton, S. E., Salmon, P., Weissbecker, L., Ulmer, C., Floyd, A., Hoover, K., Studts, J. L. K., & Studts, J. L. (2007). Mindfulness meditation alleviates depressive symptoms in women with fibromyalgia: Results of a randomized clinical trial. *Arthritis and Rheumatism, 57*(1), 77-85.

Guided Imagery
(Contributed by Vincent Bonadies)

I. Treatment Modality
Guided Imagery

II. Rationale
Imagery as a clinical intervention has been associated with a variety of physical and psychological health outcomes, such as improved mood and reduced symptoms of anxiety and depression. Research demonstrating the positive effects of guided imagery on pain and anxiety has shown that guided imagery is a versatile and flexible facilitation technique that can be used in a wide variety of settings and populations. Research also indicates that guided imagery has a positive effect with children, adults, and older adults, both male and female.

Over the past 25 years, the effectiveness of guided imagery has been increasingly established by research findings that demonstrate its positive impact on health, creativity, and performance. We now know that in many instances even ten minutes of imagery can reduce blood pressure, lower cholesterol and glucose levels in the blood, and heighten short-term immune cell activity. It can considerably reduce blood loss during surgery and morphine use after it. It lessens headaches and pain. It can accelerate weight loss and reduce anxiety, and it has been shown to reduce the aversive effects of chemotherapy, especially nausea, depression, and fatigue. The following are some research findings that demonstrate the effectiveness of guided imagery with regards to behavioral health:

A quasi-experimental design sampled 60 short-term hospitalized depressive clients, selected consecutively. The experimental group listened to a guided imagery compact disk. The Psychiatric Inpatients Comfort Scale and the Depression, Anxiety, and Stress Scales (DASS-21) were self-administered at two time points, prior to the intervention and ten days later. The Comfort and DASS-21 scales were also used in the usual care control group at these points in time. Repeated measures revealed that the treatment group had significantly improved comfort and decreased depression, anxiety, and stress over time, as compared with the controls.

A study published in the *Journal of Holistic Nursing* (Rees, 1995) showed that postpartum depression in new mothers is alleviated by guided imagery. The research with 60 first-time mothers showed that those who practiced guided imagery during the first four weeks after giving birth had less anxiety and depression and more self-esteem and confidence than their counterparts who did not use guided imagery.

III. Referrals
Clients who have been assessed and exhibit symptoms from stress, anxiety, and pain may be referred to this group. It is adaptable to most clients with behavioral health diagnoses who have the ability to follow directions and a minimal ability to think abstractly.

IV. Risk Management
Avoid clients who have severe dementia because they may be disruptive to the group. Clients who have acute psychoses should also be restricted because of their restlessness or tendency to free associate even

further. Individuals who have sexual abuse issues may feel too vulnerable in such a group, although they may also benefit from it. A discussion with such a client before the group can be helpful.

V. Structure Criteria

The Guided Imagery program will be conducted by one Certified Therapeutic Recreation Specialist for 15 to 45 minutes, depending on the length of the guided imagery script. Group size may be unlimited as long as the space is adequate. The therapist will choose a room away from noise, interruption, or any distraction. The lights may be turned down or off to decrease visual stimulation.

VI. Process Criteria

The recreational therapist will:

1. Describe guided imagery and its benefits to the clients
2. Assess the clients' previous experience with guided imagery
3. Inform the clients that guided imagery is safe and gentle, that they are always in control of the experience, and that they can leave the session silently at any time if they wish
4. Before starting the guided imagery, make sure the clients are comfortable
5. Ask clients to rate their anxiety before group on a scale of 1-10, 10 being the highest (If there are clients who want to learn guided imagery to manage pain, ask them to rate their pain on the same 10-point scale.)
6. Suggest that the clients close their eyes and begin with 5-10 minutes of deep abdominal breathing, autogenic training, or the body scan to induce a further relaxed state
7. When the clients indicate that they are completely relaxed, begin speaking or reading the guided imagery script (See sample script.)
8. When speaking or reading the guided imagery script to the clients, use a moderate tone of voice with frequent pauses
9. When the guided imagery script comes to an end, suggest to the clients to gently open their eyes
10. Allow the clients to become oriented to their surroundings (Don't be concerned if clients don't speak quickly, rather wait a few moments for the clients to respond.)
11. If the clients don't respond verbally in an appropriate amount of time, ask the clients if they would like to talk about the experience
12. If the clients wish to talk about the guided imagery experience, accept their comments in an open, non-judgmental manner
13. Some suggested questions might be: How do you feel? What did you see, smell, hear, or touch? Did the imagery convey any meaning or message to you? What did you learn from this experience and can you incorporate that into your life?
14. Another option, if the clients don't want to talk, is to suggest writing or drawing about the experience
15. Before concluding the session, ask the clients if they have any questions and if they would like to schedule another session in the future

VII. Outcome Criteria

The client will:

1. Report that anxiety has diminished on a numeric anxiety scale by 2 points or more
2. Report that pain has diminished on the numeric pain scale by 2 points or more

VIII. Credentialing

The therapist must have a demonstrated knowledge and skill in leading guided imagery and follow the facility's credentialing requirements for recreational therapists with the National Council for Therapeutic Recreation Certification.

IX. Bibliography

Apóstolo, J. L. & Kolcaba, K. (2009). The effects of guided imagery on comfort, depression, anxiety, and stress of psychiatric inpatients with depressive disorders. *Psychiatric Nursing, 23*(6).

Astin, J. A., Shapiro, S. L., & Eisenberg, D. M. (2003). Mind-body medicine: State of the science, implications for practice. *Journal of the American Board of Family Practice, 16*(2), 131-147.

Barnes, P. M., Powell-Griner, E., McFann, K., & Nahin, R. L. (2002). Complementary and alternative medicine use among adults: United States. *CDC Advance Data Report #343.*

Bonadies, V. (2009). Guided imagery as a therapeutic recreation modality to reduce pain and anxiety. *Therapeutic Recreation Journal, 43*(2), 43-55.

Beyond Ordinary Nursing. (2003). San Mateo, CA. www.integrativeimagery.com.

Dossey, B. (1995). Using imagery to help your patient heal. *American Journal of Nursing, 5,* 41-46.

Esplen, M. J., Garfinkel, P. E., Olmsted, M., Gallop, R. M., & Kennedy, S. (1998). A randomized controlled trial of guided imagery in bulimia nervosa. *Psychological Medicine, 28*(6), 1347-57.

King, J. V. (1988). A holistic technique to lower anxiety: Relaxation with guided imagery. *Journal of Holistic Nursing, 6,* 16-20.

Leja, A. N. (1989). Using guided imagery to combat postsurgical depression. *Journal of Gerontological Nursing, 15,* 7-11.

McCaffrey, R. & Taylor, N. (2005). Effective anxiety treatment prior to diagnostic cardiac catheterization. *Holistic Nursing Practitioner, 19*(2), 70-73.

Naparstek, B. (2004). *Invisible Heroes: Survivors of Trauma and How They Heal.* New York: Bantam Dell.

Pederson, C. (1995). Effect of imagery on children's pain and anxiety during cardiac catheterization. *Issues in Comprehensive Pediatric Nursing, 18*(2), 91-109.

Rees, B. L. (1995). Effect of relaxation with guided imagery on anxiety, depression, and self-esteem in Primiparas. *Journal of Holistic Nursing, 13*(3), 255-267.

Stein T. R., Olivo, E. L., Grand, S. H., Namerow, P. B., Costa, J., & Oz, M. C. (2010). A pilot study to assess the effects of a guided imagery audiotape intervention on psychological outcomes in patients undergoing coronary artery bypass graft surgery. *Holistic Nurse Practitioner, 24*(4), 213-222.

Thompson, M. B. & Coopens, N. M. (1994). The effects of guided imagery on anxiety levels and movement of clients undergoing magnetic resonance imaging. *Holistic Nursing Practice, 8,* 59-69.

Tusek, D. L., Cwynar, R., & Cosgrove, D. M. (1999). Effect of guided imagery on length of stay, pain and anxiety in cardiac surgery patients. *Journal of Cardiovascular Management, 2*, 22-28.

Utay, J. & Miller, M. (2007). Guided imagery as an effective therapeutic technique: A brief review of its history and efficacy research. *Journal of Instructional Psychology*. Retrieved January 19, 2008, from http://www.findarticles.com.

Zacharaie, R., Kristensen, J. S., Hokland, P., Ellegarrd, J., Metze, E., & Hokland, M. (1990). Effect of psychological intervention in the form of relaxation and guided imagery on cellular immune function in normal healthy subjects. *Psychotherapy and Psychosomatics, 54*, 32-39.

Reference for the body scan technique

Davis, M., Eshelman, E. R., & McKay, M. (2008). *The Relaxation and Stress Reduction Workbook*. Oakland, CA: New Harbinger Publications.

References for guided imagery scripts

Naparstek, B. (2004). *Invisible Heroes: Survivors of Trauma and How They Heal*. New York: Bantam Dell.

Naparstek, B. (1994). *Staying Well with Guided Imagery*. New York: Warner Book.

RELAXATION AND SPECIAL PLACE IMAGERY SCRIPT
(SAMPLE GUIDED IMAGERY SCRIPT)

Purpose: To reduce anxiety.

Begin by placing your body in a comfortable position, your arms and legs uncrossed, back well supported…..

Now take 3 deep breaths, allowing each breath to relax you even more…..

Let the exhalation be a letting go kind of breath, letting go of tension or discomfort…..

With each in breath, taking in what you need and with each out breath releasing anything you don't need…..

Bring your attention to the top of you head…..

Feel the scalp soften and relax and let your forehead smooth out…..

Allow all the little muscles around your eyes to soften and relax….. and let any tension flow through the cheeks as you exhale…..

Soften the muscles in your jaw…..

Imagine a wave of relaxation flowing into your neck and into your shoulders….. into your arms….. elbows….. forearms….. all the way into your hands and fingers……

Now focus on your chest, releasing any tension around your heart or lungs, relax the muscles around your ribs…..

Wrap that relaxation around your back and let a wave of relaxation travel all down the spine…..

Allow the muscles along the spine to lengthen and release…..

Soften and relax the buttocks and pelvis…..

Let the belly be very soft so that the breath moves easily down into the abdomen…..

Invite the legs to join in the relaxation now, as it moves through the thighs….. knees….. calves….. ankles….. and feet…..

Let any last bit of tension or tightness just drain out through your feet and toes…..

When you feel relaxed and comfortable let me know with a nod of your head…..

As your body remains relaxed and comfortable, imagine yourself in a very special place….. some place that is full of natural beauty, safety, and peace….. maybe a place where you have been before or it may be a place you want to create in your imagination…..

Take some time and let yourself be drawn to one place that is just right for you today…..

Let me know when you are present there…..(Wait for a response.)

Describe what it is like there…..

What do you see?…..

Are there any smells?…..

Are there any sounds?…..

What is the temperature like?.....

Where are you in this special place?…..

And how do you feel here?.....

Take some time to do whatever you would like to do here….. to relax or to do some activity…..

This is your place…..

While you are here, there might be something for you….. a message, an image, an insight, or perhaps an answer to some question you have…..

Be open to whatever is here for you…..

Remember what has been important about this experience…..

When you are ready, become aware of the current time and place…..begin to move your body…..take a deep breath, open your eyes, and feel relaxed and awake.

My Life Collage
(Contributed by Timothy James Legg)

I. Treatment Modality

My Life Collage

II. Rationale

The body of research on the use of collage therapy is relatively small. It appears to have origins in 1972 in an article by Buck and Provancher. A case study completed by Stallings (2010) demonstrated its effectiveness with older adults with dementia, concluding that the modality allowed older adults the opportunity to convey information that they may not have been otherwise capable of verbalizing. However, this can also apply to any client who may be having trouble verbalizing concerns. Collages could be shared with other members of the treatment team for additional insight and evaluation. "Unlike verbal communication, art expression is nonlinear; vastly divergent material can coexist in pictures without regard to time or context" (Cox & Cohen, 2005).

In a small study by Takata it was concluded that collage therapy without the use of time restraints fostered both self-insight and self-understanding. The author further concluded that the modality may help to promote recovery from mental health problems.

III. Referrals

This program can be used with individuals with substance-related disorders (e.g., drug or alcohol abuse) and can also be used with individuals who have mood, somatoform, factitious, dissociative, gender identity, eating, and personality disorders because of their poor communication skills, emotional distances, or lack of insight. Individuals with mild dementia or cognitive disorders who are not exhibiting acutely psychotic symptoms or disruptive behaviors may benefit.

IV. Risk Management

This program poses no extraordinary risks to the organization. The use of scissors will be monitored at all times. The therapist should count the number of pairs of scissors distributed and assure that that same number has been returned upon conclusion of the activity.

V. Structure Criteria

Sessions should be limited to one hour each to prevent fatigue and boredom. Also, clients may be scheduled to participate in other therapy groups. Depending on the depth of the collage, as well as client involvement, two or three sessions may be devoted to this activity.

VI. Process Criteria

Although individual approaches to this program may vary, the following are suggested:

Preparation of supplies

The therapist will provide a variety of magazines, non-toxic glue, safety scissors, poster-quality board, colored pencils, and non-toxic markers.

Unless the facility forbids any use of cameras, a digital camera printer-docking station is also ideal for clients who wish to include pictures of themselves in the collage. If a client currently does not want his/her picture taken, you could encourage the client to ask a family member to bring a picture from home. Pictures from home can be photocopied to preserve the original picture.

Description of Project

Once clients have been selected as appropriate for inclusion in this activity, and once the clients have agreed to participate, the therapist will describe the activity.

A sample description of this activity is as follows: "As you're aware, life is a very complicated process. More often than not, we truly lack an appreciation of everything that competes for our time and attention in life. In this exercise, we are going to have the opportunity to do just that. Today, we are going to create a collage of our lives. The rules on how to do this are very simple: Take some time to go through these magazines and, when you find a picture that represents some aspect of your life, either now, in the past, or something that you see as being instrumental to your future, cut it out. You may also use pictures of yourself today (indicate that you would be willing to take pictures of clients for use in their collages), or you can use a picture from home representing any part of your life. The good news about this project is that nobody needs to be an artist. Instead, I would like you to paint a portrait of your life using pictures, either ones found in magazines, pictures that we take, pictures that you have, or pictures that you draw. It could be your entire life; it could be a portion of your life the way it is today; it could describe some important event that happened to you in the past; or it can even tell about your dreams for the future.

The therapist can feel free to work on his/her own collage, as well. By doing this, the clients may not see themselves as an object of study, but, instead, engaging in a recreation act with the therapist who is obviously doing the project as well. The therapist should be available, however, to provide any type of technical assistance throughout the project.

Let the clients know up front that there are no "right" or "wrong" ways of preparing the collage, and that nobody will be graded on the collage, nor will anyone be mocked or criticized for his/her collage. Setting a safe zone in which the clients can feel free to express themselves is essential to achieving the therapeutic benefits of the program.

The program should also be fun-focused. Participants may wish to discuss what different images mean to them. For instance, a participant may want to share a particular memory that a given image evokes. Do not attempt to stifle that memory or discussion, as all communication can be therapeutic.

Technical assistance with the project

If a client feels that s/he needs more room, s/he can be given either a second poster board or encouraged to use the back side of the poster board.

If a client loses interest or feels that s/he has completed the collage, you may handle this in several ways. First, you can encourage the client to see what others are doing as a possible source of additional ideas, or second, you may ask the client if s/he would like another poster board to address a different aspect of his/her life. If the client wishes to leave the group, that is acceptable, as well, but be certain to note this in your progress note and follow-up with the client later. In this project, emotions may be evoked that are unpleasant or unsettling for clients. Appropriate follow-up by the recreational therapist should be undertaken.

If the collage cannot be completed in the first session, another session may be needed. Between sessions the therapist will store the projects someplace safe and should not stack them until the glue has had a sufficient chance to dry.

Once the project is completed

Once all participants have completed their collages, clients can be asked to explain the meaning of their collages to other members of the group.

The recreational therapist may ask probing questions, when or if they are appropriate. Other members of the group can ask questions and share observations, as well.

If a client chooses not to share with the group, perhaps s/he would be willing to share the description and meaning of the collage with the recreational therapist in private. This is perfectly acceptable.

Once everyone has had the opportunity to describe his/her collage, the recreational therapist should debrief the group as a whole. Questions to include in the debriefing may encompass areas such as: What did you all think of this project? Do you think that this project helped you to see any aspect of your life in a different way? If so, in what way?

Documentation

Upon completion of the project, the recreational therapist will document clients' participation in the project.

VII. Outcome Criteria

This project has three outcome criteria. Upon completion of the project, the participant will:

1. Create a collage that gives form to his/her life as s/he sees it now, describes his/her life in the past, and/or describes future goals or aspirations
2. Describe the content, arrangement, and organization of the collage in terms of what the collage represents to the client
3. Acknowledge feedback received by the therapist, counselors, psychiatrist, and other clients specific to possible meanings and observations about the overall arrangement, organization, and content of collage

VIII. Credentialing

By virtue of the fact that some sensitive areas may be touched upon as a result of this program, the program should be conducted by a Certified Therapeutic Recreation Specialist skilled in group facilitation techniques, as well as debriefing processes. Co-treatment with a licensed mental health counselor can also be considered to maximize therapeutic intervention.

IX. Bibliography

American Psychiatric Association. (2000). *Diagnostic and Statistical Manual of Mental Disorders (Fourth Edition, Text Revision)*. Washington, DC.

Buck, R. E. & Provancher, M. A. (1972). Magazine picture collage as an evaluated technique. *The American Journal of Occupational Therapy, 26*, 36-39.

Cox, C. T. & Cohen, B. M. (2005). The unique role of art making in the treatment of dissociative identity disorder. *Psychiatric Annals, 35*(8), 695-697.

Stallings, J. W. (2010). Collage as a therapeutic modality for reminiscence in patients with dementia. *Art Therapy: Journal of the American Art Therapy Association, 27*(3), 136-140.

Takata, Y. (2002). Supporting by a nurse teacher in a school infirmary using collage therapy. *Psychiatry and Clinical Neurosciences, 56*, 371-379.

Geriatric Program Protocols

The following protocols are appropriate for geriatric populations.

Morning Exercise Group

I. Treatment Modality

Morning Exercise Group

II. Rationale

The clients in an inpatient behavioral health program may range from individuals who remain ambulatory and cognitively intact to those who have an ongoing process of dementia or may be considered medically frail. Such frailty may be related to osteoporosis, arthritis, unhealed fractures or rotator cuffs, Parkinsonism, diabetes, or any number of contributing illnesses and conditions. Among this group, client falls are often a problem and programs diligently take multiple steps to prevent falls and injury. Standing exercises or even chair exercises that involve the use of the legs and feet, stretching the back of the calves and Achilles tendons, and promoting extension of joints may lead to a reduction in falls.

Among the ambulatory, "pre-frail" group of clients there often exists a malaise, lethargy, and anhedonia because of the nature of depression and anxiety which contribute, without sufficient treatment, to the physical deterioration of the individual and a decline in functional abilities in the long run. Although the intensity of exercise for this group is unlikely to produce the euphoric "runner's high," this level of exercise can be stimulating and energizing. Coupled with the social stimulation from staff attention, orientation, and the use of music or jokes, this group can produce positive mood changes.

Research studies have determined that moderate exercise benefits older persons' cardiovascular status, functional ability, mental processing (Elward & Larson, 1992), and positive behavior (Heyn et al, 2004). Such programs have proven to be safe from serious complications when they are tailored to the particular function and needs of the individuals or groups. A number of studies have demonstrated the positive effect on preventing falls in the elderly (Province et al, 1995). The use of a balance-enhancing Tai Chi-like program noted such a decline (Faber et al, 2006), and resistance training resulted in improved muscle size and strength (Evans, 1999).

The morning hours are the best time to do the exercise group. It not only is the time to wake up, but it is a good time to review the day's orientation (day, date, season, place, weather), introduce peers to one another, make announcements for the day, or plan group activities together. Music may be used as a stimulant or to set a beat for exercises. The group may end with some uplifting activity such as singing a song together, telling some clean and not-so-subtle jokes, or discussing some inspirational message.

III. Referrals

Inasmuch as anyone can benefit from an exercise program, all clients in the geriatric program may be referred by the physician for this program unless contraindicated. Reasons for referrals in a geriatric behavioral health program may include low energy levels, fatigue, depression, de-conditioning, psychomotor retardation or agitation, difficulty concentrating, or sleep disturbances.

Clients with recent or unhealed fractures may be prohibited, as well as those who have acute respiratory or other illnesses, and others whose agitated behaviors may be disruptive to the other members of the group. Individuals who have chronic respiratory illnesses may participate, depending on the medical opinion and the severity of the illness.

IV. Risk Management

There are significant concerns about risks doing physical activity with a group of clients who may be frail on admission or who are medically unstable. Even with a referring order from a physician, the therapist must be alert daily to the changeable status of clients. The therapist may notice changes in breathing, flushing, new or worsening pain, sudden weakness, especially on one side of the body, and loss of consciousness. When such severe changes are noted, the therapist will immediately ask the client to stop and notify the medical staff. When a client sustains a fall or any acute injury in the group, an incident report will be completed according to the facility's policy.

Risks to the organization and the prevention of any injury to the clients will be diminished by the proper training of the therapist in exercise and physical fitness for the elderly, including such issues as physical assessment, proper techniques in exercise and use of equipment, and fall prevention.

V. Structure Criteria

The recreational therapist will conduct this group in the mornings daily for 45 minutes in a space that is large enough and unencumbered by obstacles that may present a risk of falls. Music may be used at times to stimulate energy, but should be turned off when clients are introducing themselves.

Members of the group are encouraged to participate to the best of their ability, and if they have pain, they may cease participation in all or part of the exercises.

VI. Process Criteria

The therapist begins by welcoming participants to the group. Members, seated in a circle, take turns introducing themselves by first name to the group. In order to build connections with one another in the group, participants may also be asked to respond to a common question or theme, such as: What do you like to do in the winter? Or what sort of work did you do?

The therapist will introduce the group's activities of the day. Each day the therapist may discuss a different idea in the process of the group, such as the benefits of exercise on physical health, the importance of exercise for fall prevention, or the significance of exercise in reducing depression and anxiety.

The group begins with about 10 minutes of warm-ups. This may be light stretches or bouncing and throwing a ball around the circle.

The therapist then leads the group in approximately 25 minutes of stretching exercises or the use of stretch bands. If any exercises are performed from a standing position, only persons who are ambulatory without assistive walkers or canes will be included. A chair must be within easy reach for a client to reach out and hold for balance, if needed.

Ten minutes of cool-down movement or diaphragmatic breathing exercises will complete the program. During the final moments, the therapist will ask the group members to identify the day, date, year, and where they currently are. Finally, the therapist may use this time to make announcements about the day's schedule, discuss the visiting hours, or make plans together for other activities. During this time the group may want to sing familiar songs together, or the therapist may engage the group by telling jokes.

VII. Outcome Criteria

Clients may anticipate improvements following participation in this Morning Exercise program such as these outcomes:

1. Improved alertness for the length of the group
2. Improved concentration with no more than one or two prompts from the therapist
3. Increased energy throughout the day
4. Being able to repeat the day's orientation information
5. Increased awareness of others in group
6. Being able to explain the benefits of exercise on fall prevention and recovery from depression and anxiety

VIII. Credentialing

The therapist will hold certification from the National Council for Therapeutic Recreation Certification, have demonstrated expertise in fitness, knowledge of medical illness and complications in the elderly, and follow the facility's requirements for minimum qualifications and credentialing.

IX. Bibliography

American Psychiatric Association. (2000). *Diagnostic and Statistical Manual of Mental Disorders (Fourth Edition, Text Revision)*. Washington, DC.

Buettner, L. & Fitzsimmons, S. (2003). *Dementia Practice Guidelines for Recreational Therapy: Treatment of Disturbing Behaviors*. Alexandria, VA: American Therapeutic Recreation Association.

Conn, V. S., Valentine, J. C., & Cooper, H. M. (2002). Interventions to increase physical activity among older adults: A meta-analysis. *Annals of Behavioral Medicine, 24*(3), 190-200.

Dishman, R. K. (1994). Motivating older adults to exercise. *Southern Medical Journal, 87*, S79-82.

Elward, K. & Larson, E. B. (1992). Benefits of exercise for older adults: A review of existing evidence and current recommendations for the general population. *Clinics in Geriatric Medicine, 8*(1), 35-50.

Evans, W. J. (1999). Exercise training guidelines for the elderly. *Medicine and Science in Sports and Exercise, 31*(1), 12-17.

Faber, M. J., Bosscher, R. J., Paw, M. J., & Van Wieringen, P. C. (2006). Effects of exercise programs on falls and mobility in frail and pre-frail older adults: A multicenter randomized controlled trial. *Archives of Physical Medicine and Rehabilitation, 87*(7), 885-896.

Fitzsimmons, S. & Buettner, L. L. (2009). The recreational therapist's role in treating delirium. *American Journal of Recreation Therapy, 8*(1), 33-47.

Gill, T. M. & Allore, H. (2002). A program to prevent functional decline in physically frail, elderly persons who live at home. *The New England Journal of Medicine, 347*, 1068-1074.

Heath, J. M. & Stuart, M. R. (2002). Prescribing exercise for frail elders. *Journal of the American Board of Family Medicine, 15*(3), 218-228.

Heyn, P., Abreu, B. C., & Ottenbacher, K. J. (2004). The effects of exercise training on elderly persons with cognitive impairment and dementia: A meta-analysis. *Archives of Physical Medicine and Rehabilitation, 85*(10), 1694-1704.

Netz, Y., Wu, M-J., Becker, B. J., & Tenenbaum, G. (2005). Physical activity and psychological well-being in advanced age: A meta-analysis of intervention studies. *Psychology and Aging, 20*(2), 272-284.

Province, M. A., et al (1995). The effects of exercise on falls in elderly patients. *JAMA, 273*(17), 1341-1347.

Rolland, Y., Pillard, F., Klapouszcak, A., Reynish, E., Thomas, D., Andrieu, S., & Vellas, B. (2007). Exercise program for nursing home residents with Alzheimer's disease: A 1-year randomized, controlled trial. *Journal of the American Geriatrics Society, 55*(2), 158-165.

Williams, C. L. & Tappen, R. M. (2007). Effect of exercise on mood in nursing home residents with Alzheimer's disease. *American Journal of Alzheimer's Disease and Other Dementias, 22*, 389-397.

Woodhead, E. L., Zarit, S. H., Braungart, E. R., Rovine, M. R., & Femia, E. E. (2005). Behavioral and psychological symptoms of dementia: The effects of physical activity at adult day centers. *American Journal of Alzheimer's Disease and Other Dementias, 20*, 171.

Octaband® Movement
(Contributed by Donna Neuman-Bluestein)

I. Treatment Modality

Octaband® Movement

The Octaband® is a motivational tool for expressive movement and socialization.

II. Rationale

Dementia of the Alzheimer's type, vascular, or due to other general medical conditions is characterized by the presence of multiple cognitive deficits including decline in attention and concentration. These cognitive deficits also cause significant impairment in social or occupational functioning.

Additionally, according to the Surgeon General's report, between "8 and 20 percent of older adults in the community and up to 37 percent in primary care settings suffer from depressive symptoms…. The diagnosis of minor depression is not yet standardized; the research criteria proposed in *DSM-IV-TR* are the same as those for major depression, but a diagnosis would require fewer symptoms and less impairment."

Exercise has proven physical, cognitive, and emotional benefits for older adults. In a study with people with late-stage dementia, Dayanim (2009) found that participation in a 20-minute expressive movement group led to a statistically significant decrease in clients' aphasia and/or agnosia and memory recall following the program. Shustik and Thompson (2001) reported that core psychological needs of persons with dementia may be met through movement dialogue and communication that occur through the use of a stretch cloth, with each member of the group holding the material.

In their 2003 study, Verghese et al. found that dancing was the only physical activity associated with a lower risk of dementia.

People with dementia often lose concentration and wander off during activities. In their study, Dr. Susan Ruka and Dody Coman (2009) found that people with dementia will hang on to the hemmed ends of the Octaband® and lift longer than they will sustain an interest in returning a ball in a ball toss.

III. Referrals

Older adults with mid- to late-stage dementia and/or depressive symptoms may be referred to this program if they exhibit any or all of the following:

1. Diminished ability to concentrate
2. Social isolation
3. Depressed mood
4. Diminished interest or pleasure in most activities
5. Insomnia
6. Psychomotor agitation or retardation
7. Feelings of worthlessness

There should be no contraindications based on physical functioning and no tendency to become overstimulated.

IV. Risk Management

Participants will be observed to determine that safe exercise procedures are followed. Activity will be monitored at all times. Any injuries will be reported immediately to the appropriate nursing and/or medical staff and an incident report will be completed. Since exercise with the Octaband® is not overly strenuous, there is not likely to be significant risk to the clients or the organization. Clients will be instructed to remain seated, since they could become entangled in the arms of the Octaband® if they are attempting to walk through it.

V. Structure Criteria

The Octaband® program is to be conducted for at least 50 minutes once weekly in a recreation space free of tables, 8 to 12 feet in diameter. Ideal group size is between 6 and 16 participants. Participants will be seated in a circle.

VI. Process Criteria

The recreational therapist will screen all participants to ensure there are no contraindications based on physical functioning or a tendency to become overstimulated.

5-minute preparation

1. The recreational therapist will offer and respect the choice of each person in the circle in regards to holding an Octaband® leg.
2. The recreational therapist will sequentially slip the loop at the end of each leg over the wrist of each participant sitting in the circle.
3. If the older adult chooses not to hold an Octaband® leg, but is willing, the recreational therapist may tie a leg of the Octaband® onto the arm of the participant's chair or wheelchair.

15-minute warm-up exercise

The therapist will

1. Play rhythmic music familiar to participants based on age and culture, or sing the refrain of a familiar song, such as "Hello Dolly" or "Once in Love with Amy," replacing the name "Amy" with the name of each person in the group.
2. Make small bouncy movements in time to the music, picking up on participants' rhythms if possible.
3. Name each member of the group, asking each to demonstrate a movement for all to mirror.
4. Suggest that participants stretch arms, reaching up and in as many directions and as far as possible.
5. Name each part of the body from head to toe and suggest that participants move using self-touch as much as possible.
6. Encourage participants to shake arms to release tension.

7. Encourage participants to hold the Octaband® low, as each person attempts to stretch one leg over the Octaband® leg. Repeat with other leg.

The following exercises will be led by the therapist:

8. Gently swing arms from side to side.
9. Cross both arms in front and then out to the sides.
10. Gently bring one arm up while bringing the other arm down.
11. Lift one arm up diagonally across the body and bring it down. Repeat with the other arm.
12. Pull on the legs, bending elbows, and release, extending arms.
13. Alternative ways of moving initiated by participants will be invited and welcomed by the recreation therapist and integrated into the session in the moment.

5-minute breathing with movement exercise

The recreational therapist will demonstrate breathing coordinated with movement as everyone raises arms up on the inhale and brings arms down on the exhale.

15-minute exercise bouncing weighted objects in the center of the Octaband®

1. The recreational therapist will place a weighted object, such as a beanbag or ball, on the Octaband®. If the group does well, up to eight such weighted objects may be used.
2. The therapist will encourage bouncing the object on the Octaband®, attempting to keep it in the center.
3. If participants are doing well, the therapist may count the number of successful bounces without dropping the object, each time trying to improve over the last best score.
4. To recuperate from their focused attention, participants can then see how quickly they can shake all the objects off.

5-minute group dance

1. The recreational therapist will play Big Band music or any other uplifting music.
2. The therapist will follow the impulse of individual group members, suggesting that others do the same.

5-minute cool down

1. The recreational therapist will play slow music to encourage greater relaxation.
2. The therapist will encourage the members to coordinate their breaths with the movement: everyone raises their arms on the inhale and brings their arms down on the exhale.

VII. Outcome Criteria

The older adult will:

1. Work cooperatively with other group members to accomplish the tasks
2. Experience prolonged concentration throughout the group

3. Exhibit increased spontaneity and more interactions, including coherent verbalizations
4. Exhibit improved affect through more frequent smiles
5. Demonstrate increased awareness of others
6. Report feeling calm at the conclusion

VIII. Credentialing

The recreational therapist leading this program will be certified by the National Council for Therapeutic Recreation Certification as a CTRS. The program may also be led or co-led by a Dance/Movement Therapist registered with the American Dance Therapy Association or board-certified by the Dance/Movement Therapy Certification Board. Therapists will be knowledgeable of safety issues in the geriatric population.

IX. Bibliography

American Psychiatric Association. (2000). *Diagnostic and Statistical Manual of Mental Disorders (Fourth Edition, Text Revision)*. Washington, DC.

Dayanim, S. (2009). The acute effects of a specialized movement program on the verbal abilities of patients with late-state dementia. *Alzheimer's Care Today, 10*(2), 93-98.

Mental Health: A Report of the Surgeon General. http://www.surgeongeneral.gov/library/mentalhealth/chapter5/sec3.html#diagnosis. (Retrieved November 5, 2011).

Ruka, S. & Coman, D. (2009). *Octaband® increases engagement in elders with dementia*. Merriman House-Memorial Hospital Internal Quality Assurance Research.

Shustik, L. R. & Thompson, T. (2001). Dance/movement therapy: Partners in personhood. In A. Innes & K. Hatfield (Eds.). *Healing Arts Therapies and Person-centered Dementia Care*. London: Jessica Kingsley.

Verghese, J., Lipton, R. B., Katz, M. J., Hall, C. B., Derby, C. A., Kuslansky, G., Ambrose, A. F., Sliwinski, M., & Buschke, H. (2003). Leisure activities and the risk of dementia in the elderly. *New England Journal of Medicine, 348*, 2508-2516.

Garden Group
(Contributed by Wendy Maran)

I. Treatment Modality

Garden Group

II. Rationale

Clients that are treated for geriatric psychiatric issues present with a wide variety of impairments. These impairments include, but are not limited to, short- and long-term memory deficits; deficits associated with abstract thinking, sequencing, judgment, and recognition; problems with objects and individuals; disorientation; anxiety; agitation; language problems; and motor deficits.

Gardening produces an opportunity to exercise naturally in a stress-relieving, rewarding activity. It is a rewarding leisure pursuit that produces a natural avenue to work on all major muscle groups and joints, full range of motion, and fine motor work as well (Rothert, 1994). Gardening, for many, is a pastime that brought great satisfaction and enjoyment pre-morbidly and should be used as a success-oriented therapeutic modality.

There is research that suggests that horticulture and gardening as a therapy provides a safe, non-threatening environment that can reduce agitation and anxiety. It provides opportunities for sensory stimulation and reminiscence, increases attention span, and increases opportunities for functional skill practice. Pairing the activity with the season or event helps decrease confusion (Hewson, 1995). Gardening activities are highly adaptable and provide a wide variety of activities for many different levels of functioning. These activities can promote carryover of skills to increase independence and functioning in activities of daily living (ADLs). Gardening and garden-based activities offer many challenges for the body and mind, provide an opportunity to be creative and practice skills from simple to complex, and are very forgiving pursuits where you can do it your way without much problem (Rothert, 1994). Studies that have been conducted on people and plant interactions suggest there is a profound effect on human well being through passive and active participation in the natural environment with plants (Barnicle and StoelzleMidden, 2011).

Through observation of clients in garden activities, therapists can identify problem behaviors such as isolative behavior, socially inappropriate behavior, inability to work independently and or cooperatively, and cognition level. The activity needs to be congruent with the clients' ability level and be tailored to the symptoms that the clients are experiencing on the day they are to participate (Hewson, 1995). Gardening is a very functional, success-oriented modality.

III. Referrals

Garden Group is open to anyone who is interested in working with horticulture material. All clients should be invited but allowed to refuse if they do not want to go to group. If the client is demonstrating behaviors that would be contraindicated (e.g., actively hallucinating), s/he may not participate in garden group during that time. The therapist will assess the client's ability to participate each day.

IV. Risk Management

Risks associated with horticulture/gardening activities can be little or great depending on the individual.

Potential reactions to plants, insects, and other environmental risks must be known. It is important that the therapist knows the client's allergies prior to involvement in gardening activities. Always have first aid equipment on hand and know procedures that are needed for clients that may have reactions to insect bites. Offer gloves to your clients. It should be their choice if they wish to use them. Practice good hand washing techniques when finished in the garden to decrease transfer of irritants as well as maintaining cleanliness. To minimize risk, work with non-poisonous plant material whenever possible. The Joint Commission requires that all indoor house plants be non-toxic (Joint Commission, 2011). Inform your clients about the plants that they are working with. There are websites and many books that list poisonous plants, if the therapist is unsure. Always consult resources if there is a question about the safety of a particular plant. If a client has a habit of placing things in his/her mouth, consider having the client wear a mask. This will also reduce the possibility of inhaling irritants from plants and flowers. Consider using visual aids, like picture cards or cue cards, to help connect the client to the task and the plants that may pose a risk. (Hewson, 1995).

Garden tools and shears may be sharp. Staff will closely supervise clients in their use and make sure that all tools are returned at the end of the session.

V. Structure Criteria

The Garden Group will meet three times a week for 60 minutes. The group will be outside in the garden area when weather permits. During the winter or inclement weather the Garden Group will meet in the recreational therapy room or indoor gardening room.

A wide variety of gardening activities will involve the clients in a variety of tasks that can enhance and promote retention of skills. Tasks may involve the following areas:

Physical Functioning

Clients may improve gross and fine motor skills, build and maintain endurance, coordination, and strength, and promote overall well-being through such tasks as planting, weeding, fertilizing, harvesting, and the use of adaptive tools that are complementary to the functioning level and ability of the client.

Cognitive

Memory, concentration, attention, reality orientation, and sensory stimulation can all be enhanced by involvement in the maintenance tasks associated with garden group programs such as planning, using watering schedules, plant propagation, transplanting, cultivating the plants and flowers, and crafts that involve garden material.

Social Emotional

Garden activities naturally create an environment to work on social interaction skills through rapport-building activities, cooperation skills, planning, and organizing. Involvement in familiar success-oriented activities increases self-esteem and feelings of self-worth while decreasing anxiety.

VI. Process Criteria

The therapist will:

1. Prepare the room or area for the activity if needed
2. Invite the chosen clients to participate in the garden activity
3. Demonstrate how to do the activity
4. Assist the client in use of the items for the activity
5. Be alert to possible safety risks

Physical

1. Assist the client in choosing the correct tool for the activity
2. Help the client compensate for personal physical limitations when participating in the garden activity
3. Demonstrate and instruct the clients in the activity

Cognitive

1. Assist the client in developing maintenance schedules for watering, weeding, deadheading, and general garden care
2. Assist the client in the sequencing steps of the garden activity
3. Help the clients to identify plants, flowers, and other garden items

Social/Emotional

1. Facilitate the clients interaction with peers and therapists in a positive manner
2. Demonstrate and instruct the clients in garden crafts and activities
3. Assist the clients in identifying feelings associated with the activity

VII. Outcome Criteria

Physical

1. The client will actively participate in the garden tasks to his/her full ability
2. The client will use adapted techniques or tools with or without assistance

Cognitive

1. The client will perform garden maintenance tasks with or without reminders and assistance
2. The client will demonstrate increased executive functioning with tasks
3. The client will be able to identify a wide variety of plants and garden items

Social/Emotional

1. The client will interact in a positive and cooperative manner with peers and staff
2. The client will show increased self-esteem and feelings of self-worth
3. The client will demonstrate less anxiety

VIII. Credentialing

There should be at a minimum one CTRS (certified by the National Council for Therapeutic Recreation Certification) involved in each session. The CTRS should have knowledge of gardening and plants. Some additional training or certification in using plants as a therapeutic medium would be advised but not mandatory. If the CTRS does not have gardening experience, then there should be a volunteer or alternate staff member with gardening experience in addition to the CTRS for every session.

IX. Bibliography

Adil, J. (1994). *Accessible Gardening for People with Physical Disabilities: A Guide to Methods, Tools, and Plants*. Ravensdale, WA: Idyll Arbor.

Aggie Horticulture. AgriLife Extension: Texas A & M System. www.aggie-horticulture.tamu.edu/lawn_garden/poison/poison.html. Retrieved 12/23/11.

American Horticulture Therapy Association Definitions and Positions. http://www.ahta.org/sitefiles/sitepages/c2c40f8e313a7002afab8d46beb97636.pdf. Retrieved 12/18/2011.

Banzinger, G. & Rousch, S. (1983). Nursing homes for the birds: A control-relevant intervention with bird feeders. *The Gerontologist, 23*, 527-531.

Barnicle, T. & StoelzleMidden, K. The effects of a horticulture activity program on the psychological well-being of older people in a long-term care facility. http://horttech.ashspublications.org/content/13/1/81.full.pdf. Retrieved 12/19/2011.

Hewson, M. (1995). *Horticulture as Therapy: A Practical Guide to Using Horticulture as a Therapeutic Tool*. Ravensdale, WA: Idyll Arbor, Inc.

The Joint Commission. http://www.jointcommission.org/standards_information/standards.aspx. Retrieved 12/26/2011.

Poisonous Plants Home Page. University of Pennsylvania. www.cal.vet.upenn.edu/projects/poison/index.html. Retrieved 12/23/11.

Rothert, G. (1994). *Enabling Garden: Creating Barrier-Free Gardens*. Dallas, TX: Taylor Publishing Company.

Leisure Education

I. Treatment Modality

Leisure Education

II. Rationale

Many of the clients who are admitted to a geriatric behavioral health program have ineffective or insufficient patterns of participation in leisure activities. Those with depression or anxiety may have past interests but no recent record of involvement because of a decreased interest in pleasurable activities. Those with thought disorders such as schizophrenia or schizoaffective disorders may lack the necessary social skills to develop social contacts that support participation in expressed interests. Those with a manic episode of a bipolar disorder lack the focus to attend to their interests for periods of time without excessive behaviors. Finally, clients who have dementia experience a lack of initiative to independently and safely engage in meaningful activity. Disruptive behaviors often occur among these clients when they do not feel a sense of purposeful activity. All of these clients may benefit from structured modalities that are planned to meet their particular interests, skills, and cognitive abilities, to be stimulating and engaging but not over-challenging. In addition, there is a growing body of literature which suggests that the amount and quality of leisure-time activities that one participates in is inversely associated with the development of dementias.

III. Referrals

Clients may be referred to a leisure education program if they exhibit any of the diagnoses discussed above, unless their behaviors are disruptive to the group process. Careful attention will be taken by the recreational therapist to place individuals in groups of other clients with whom they may be compatible. For instance, a client who is cognitively intact may not wish to be in a group with many clients who have advanced dementia and, therefore, may not benefit from the treatment group.

IV. Risk Management

Since the scope of possible modalities used in the Leisure Education program can be very broad, it is difficult to judge all possible risks. It is important that the therapist maintains watchful supervision when sharp implements are being used or when clients might ingest substances like dirt or fertilizer in a gardening program. When using craft supplies, the therapist will use only non-toxic glues, markers, or paints.

V. Structure Criteria

The Leisure Education group will meet daily for up to one hour, although some groups of clients may be able to tolerate only shorter periods of time. The room should be well lit with ample room for the activities. Modalities will be chosen to meet the assessed needs of the client group and from among expressed interests from the clients. Examples of modalities may include active games, board games, arts and crafts, music, cooking, and gardening.

VI. Process Criteria

The therapist will introduce the clients in the group to the modality for the day, or, if the clients are able to make a decision together, offer the group a choice of several modalities. In the beginning the therapist may need to provide some instruction to introduce the modality. Throughout the group, the therapist will provide supervision for any potential risks. All clients will be encouraged to participate according to their abilities. Assistance will be provided to the client upon request, but the therapist will resist efforts to take over for the client. When this occurs, it's usually because the activity chosen is too difficult for the client. At this point the activity may be modified so that the client can have more success. There are times when a more able client may be paired with and offer assistance to a peer who needs more assistance. If any client's behavior in the group becomes disruptive, the therapist will use behavioral management strategies to refocus the client's attention back to the task, if that is possible. When the behavior cannot be changed with redirecting techniques, the therapist may suggest that it is better for the client to leave the room because it is too stimulating.

VII. Outcome Criteria

At the conclusion of the group, the client will be able to:

1. Attend to the task at hand for a minimum of 30, 45, or 60 minutes
2. Demonstrate successful participation in the activity according to the client's ability level
3. Report enjoyment of activity
4. Not demonstrate disruptive behaviors that interfere with the client's participation or the group process
5. Participate in activities that the client may be able to engage in later at home

VIII. Credentialing

The therapist will be a Certified Therapeutic Recreation Specialist (CTRS) certified by the National Council for Therapeutic Recreation Certification and will be skilled in the leadership of a wide variety of recreational modalities.

IX. Bibliography

Abraham, C. & Michie, S. (2008). A taxonomy of behavior change techniques used in interventions. *Health Psychology, 27*(3), 379-387.

Buettner, L. & Fitzsimmons, S. (2003). *Dementia Practice Guideline for Recreational Therapy: Treatment of Disturbing Behaviors.* Alexandria, VA: American Therapeutic Recreation Association.

Buettner, L., Fitzsimmons, S., & Atav, S. (2006). Predicting outcomes of therapeutic recreation interventions for older adults with dementia and behavior symptoms. *Therapeutic Recreation Journal, 40,* 33-47.

Coyle, C. P., Kinney, W. B., Riley, R., & Shank, J. (eds.) (1991). *Benefits of Therapeutic Recreation: A Consensus View.* Ravensdale, WA: Idyll Arbor, Inc.

Kolanowski, A. M., Buettner, L., Costa, P. T. Jr., & Litaker, M. S. (2001). Capturing interests: Therapeutic recreation activities for persons with dementia. *Therapeutic Recreation Journal, 35*(3), 220-235.

Fabrigoule, C., Letenneru L., Dartigues, J. F., Zarrouk, M., & Commenges, D. (1995). Social and leisure activities and risk of dementia: A prospective longitudinal study. *Journal of the American Geriatrics Society, 43*, 485-490.

Fritsch, T., Smyth, K. A., Debanne, S. M., Petot, G. J., & Friedland, R. P. (2005). Participation in novelty-seeking leisure activities and Alzheimer's disease. *Journal of Geriatric Psychiatry and Neurology, 18*, 134-141.

Harmer, B. J. & Orrell, M. (2008). What is meaningful activity for people with dementia living in care homes? A comparison of the views of older people with dementia, staff and family carers. *Aging and Mental Health, 12*(5), 548-558.

Langer, E. J. & Rodin, J. (1976). The effects of choice and enhanced personal responsibility for the aged: A field experiment in an institutional setting. *Journal of Personality and Social Psychology, 34*, 191-198.

Mahoney, A. E. J. (2003). Age or stage-appropriate? Recreation and the relevance of Piaget's theory in dementia care. *American Journal of Alzheimer's Disease and Other Dementias, 18*, 24-30.

Myllykangas, S. A., Gosselink, C. A., Foose, A. K., & Gaede, D. B. (2002). Meaningful activity in older adults: Being in flow. *World Leisure Journal, 44*, 24-33.

Podewills, L. J., Gualler, E., Kuller, L. H., Fired, L. P., Lopez, O. L., Carlson, M., et al. (2005). Physical activity, APOE genotype, and dementia risk: Findings from the cardiovascular health cognition study. *American Journal of Epidemiology, 161*, 639-651.

Russoniello, C. V. (1991). An exploratory study of physiological and psychological changes in alcoholic clients after recreation therapy treatments. Paper presented at the Benefits of Therapeutic Recreation in Rehabilitation Conference, Lafayette Hill, PA.

Scarmeas, N., Levy, G., Tang, M. X., Manly, J., & Stern, Y. (2001). Influence of leisure activity on the incidence of Alzheimer's disease. *Neurology, 57*, 2236-2242.

Schreiner, A. S., Yamomoto, E., & Shiotani, H. (2005). Positive affect among nursing home residents with Alzheimer's dementia: The effect of recreational activity. *Aging & Mental Health, 9*(2), 129-134.

Schooler, C. & Mulatu, M. S. (2001). The reciprocal effects of leisure time activities and intellectual functioning in older people: A longitudinal analysis. *Psychology and Aging, 16*, 466-482.

Tortosa-Martinez, J., Zoerink, D. A., & Yoder, D. G. (2011). The benefits of therapeutic recreation experiences for people with Alzheimer's disease. *Annual in Therapeutic Recreation, 19*, 52-65.

Wang, H. X., Karp, A., Winbad, B., & Fratiglioni, L. (2002). Late-life engagement in social and leisure activities is associated with a decreased risk of dementia: A longitudinal study from the Kungsholmen project. *American Journal of Epidemiology, 155*, 1081-1087.

Wong, S. E., Terranova, M. D., Marshall, B. D., Banzett, L. K., & Liberman, R. P. (1983). Reducing bizarre stereotypic behavior in chronic psychiatric clients: Effects of supervised and independent recreational activities. Presented at the Ninth Annual Convention of the Association of Behavior Analysis, Milwaukee, WI.

Aromatherapy

I.   Treatment Modality

Aromatherapy

II.   Rationale

Clients are treated in geriatric mental health units for a variety of antisocial and difficult behaviors that accompany the diagnosis of dementia. These behaviors may range from mild anxiety to severe agitation and sun-downing. These may be difficult to address without the use of medications that may be sedating and may increase the client's risk of falling. Other issues that present with the clients include loss of appetite, poor sleep, pain, and lethargy. Pharmacological treatments may not be as effective as needed or may produce undesirable side effects. One non-pharmacological intervention that may be helpful in reducing the incidence and severity of such behaviors is the use of essential oil aromatherapy.

There is a growing body of literature which suggests the efficacious use of aromatherapy to address difficult behaviors in the elderly. One of the most rigorous studies (Kiecolt-Glaser et al, 2008) found clear evidence that lemon oil inhalation increased positive mood and also increased the release of norepinephrine, a neurotransmitter which is lowered in those with depression. In Japan, rosemary and lemon oils in the morning and lavender and orange oils in the evening were responsible for a significant improvement in overall cognitive functioning among 28 subjects. Lemon balm, also known as *Melissa*, reduced agitation when applied to the face (Ballard et al, 2002). A blend of aromatherapy called *Restore Peace* (frankincense and grapefruit oils), when used in two long-term care facilities in Texas, was credited with reducing disruptive behaviors from 1718 to 604 incidents in one month (Farnell, 2006). During an eight-month period at the Mattie C. Hall Health Care Center in South Carolina, there was a decline in weight loss of three pounds or more by using grapefruit oil (Farnell, 2006).

A number of studies combined the use of aromatherapy with hand massage. The results are statistically significant for positive outcomes, however the combination makes it difficult to determine the tools responsible for the outcomes. In England (Smallwood et al, 2001), this combination with lavender oil was used in a randomly assigned study and was effective for reducing excessive motor behavior in the afternoon. A second study from England (Kilstoff & Chenoweth, 1998) used a combination of distillation of *lavender angustifolia* and hand massage in a controlled trial with 15 daycare subjects with dementia over eighteen months. Staff and home care givers reported improvements in health and well being for subjects, more alertness, reduced agitation, and improved nighttime sleep in 60% of the subjects.

Lavender was also used in Japan (Fujii et al, 2008) with 28 subjects with moderate to severe dementia. The oil was applied to the clothing of the subjects to produce a significant reduction of hallucinations, agitation/aggression, and irritability/lability.

III.   Referrals

This program is particularly designed for clients who are diagnosed with any form of dementia. Nevertheless, any client who wishes to participate in the program would be permitted unless s/he has known allergies to an essential oil.

IV. Risk Management

Overall, essential oils carry little risk, but there are precautions to take. Aromatherapy oils must be designated as "pure" essential oils in order to verify the proper concentration for usefulness. Few side effects are noted in the literature, but they should not be applied "neat," meaning directly on bare skin. They should be used along with some unscented lotion.

Although reactions are unlikely, if a client develops a skin rash or any breathing difficulty, the oils should be stopped immediately. If a rash does appear, washing the area with soap and water will diminish it. Oils that are inhaled do not metabolize in the liver (Buckle, 2005), and thus may pose the lowest risk overall.

Using aromatherapy oils in consultation with a trained aromatherapist can mitigate any concerns.

V.   Structure Criteria

Aromatherapy will be used in individual sessions with clients. Prior to beginning the session, the therapist will seek a medical order to use aromatherapy.

The therapist will decide which difficult behaviors in the clients the aromatherapy is targeted to ameliorate. For example, a blend of frankincense and grapefruit may decrease the incidence of late afternoon agitated behaviors that are often called "sun-downing." Lavender, vetiver, and bergamot may promote sleep at night. Sandalwood, lemon balm (*Melissa*), and jasmine may promote relaxation and relief from stress.

The effects of the oils should occur within a few minutes and do not require successive applications to enhance the effect. Each session should last about 15 minutes.

VI. Process Criteria

The therapist will:

1. Invite the client to engage in the use of aromatherapy
2. Encourage the client to smell the oil prior to use
3. Explain what the use of the oils is intended to improve
4. Respect the client's right to refuse the use of the oils
5. In the presence of the client, place a drop or two of the oil in the hand with a small amount of unscented hand lotion
6. Massage the oil/lotion onto the client's hands using gentle movements
7. At the end of the hand massage, encourage the client to breathe in the scent from his/her hands

VII. Outcome Criteria

As a result of the intervention, the client may, depending on the oils used and the purpose for which they are used:

1. Report improved mood
2. Report a sense of calm
3. Demonstrate observable reductions in agitation or restlessness
4. Be able to fall asleep and remain asleep for longer periods of time

VIII. Credentialing

The therapist who uses aromatherapy must have a knowledge of aromatherapy research, how to use it properly, and what risks to anticipate. The facility may wish to have the consultation of a trained aromatherapist to support the staff in the use of the oils.

IX. Bibliography

Akhondzadeh, S. M., Noroozian, M., Mohammadi, S., Ohadinia, A., Jamshidi, H., & Khani, M. (2003). *Salvia officinalis* extract in the treatment of patients with mild to moderate Alzheimer's disease: A double-blind, randomized and placebo-controlled trial. *Journal of Clinical Pharmacy and Therapeutics, 28*, 53-59.

Ballard, C. G., Gauthier, S., Cummings, J. L., Brodaty, H., Grossberg, G. T., Robert, P., & Lyketsos, C. G. (2009). Management of agitation and aggression associated with Alzheimer's disease. *Nature Reviews/Neurology, 5*, 245-255.

Ballard, C. G., O'Brien, J. T., Reichelt, K., & Perry, E. K. (2002). Aromatherapy as a safe and effective treatment for the management of agitation in severe dementia: The results of a double-blind, placebo-controlled trial with *Melissa*. *Journal of Clinical Psychiatry, 63*, 553-558.

Baser, K. H. C. & Buchbauer, G. (2010). *Handbook of Essential Oils: Science, Technology and Applications*. Boca Raton: CRC Press.

Buckle, J. (2003). *Clinical Aromatherapy: Essential Oils in Practice*, 2nd ed. London: Churchill Livingstone.

Cuba, R. (2000). Toxicity myths — The actual risks of essential oil use. *The International Journal of Aromatherapy, 10*(2), 37-49.

Farnell, J. (2006). *Scents-ible Solutions Aromatherapy Program: Training Manual*. Aiken, SC.

Fujii, M., Hatakeyama, R., Fukuoka, Y., Yamamoto, T., Sasaki, R., Moriya, M., Kanno, M., & Sasaki, H. (2008). Lavender aroma therapy for behavioral and psychological symptoms in dementia patients. *Geriatric Gerontology International, 8*, 236-238.

Holmes, C., Hopkins, V., Hensford, C., MacLaughlin, V., Wilkinson, D., & Rosenvinge, H. (2002). Lavender oil as a treatment for agitated behaviour in severe dementia: A placebo controlled study. *International Journal of Geriatric Psychiatry, 17*, 305-308.

Jimbo, D., Kimura, Y., Taniguchi, M., Inoue, M., & Urakami, K. (2009). Effect of aromatherapy on patients with Alzheimer's disease. *Psychogeriatrics, 9*, 173-179.

Kiecolt-Glaser, J. K., Graham, J. E., Malarkey, W. B., Porter, K., Lemeshow, S., & Glaser, R. (2008). Olfactory influences on mood and autonomic, endocrine, and immune function. *Psychoneuroendocrinology, 33*(3), 328-339.

Kilstoff, K. & Chenoweth, L. (1998). New approaches to health and well-being for dementia day-care clients, family carers and day-care staff. *International Journal of Nursing Practice, 4*, 70-83.

Lis-Balchin, M. (2006). *Aromatherapy science: a guide for healthcare professionals*. London: Pharmaceutical Press.

Nguyen, Q. & Patan, C. (2008). The use of aromatherapy to treat behavioural problems in dementia. *International Journal of Geriatric Psychiatry, 23*, 337-346.

Opie, J., Rosenwarne, R., & O'Connor, D. W. (1999). The efficacy of psychosocial approaches to behaviors disorders in dementia: A systematic literature review. *Australian and New Zealand Journal of Psychiatry, 33*, 789-799.

Resnick, B. (2003). Putting research into practice: Behavioral and pharmacologic management of dementia. *Geriatric Nursing, 24*(1), 58-59.

Smallwood, J., Brown, R., Coulter, F., Irvine, E., & Copland, C. (2001). Aromatherapy and behaviour disturbances in dementia: A randomized controlled trial. *International Journal of Geriatric Psychiatry, 16*, 1010-1013.

Yim, V. W. C., Ng, A. K. Y., Tsang, H. W. H., & Leung, A. Y. (2009). A review on the effects of aromatherapy for patients with depressive symptoms. *The Journal of Alternative and Complementary Medicine, 15*(2), 187-195.

Cognitive Stimulation

I.   Treatment Modality

Cognitive Stimulation

II.   Rationale

Remaining mentally fit is a lifelong process which begins in childhood and progresses through old age. The scientific study of neuroplasticity informs us that our brains can continue to create new brains cells and new brain "maps" throughout our lives, although more slowly in older years. Those people with more brain reserves may begin to develop dementia, but, because they have more brain cells to spare, they may show few signs of the illness.

In geriatric behavioral health programs, there is a large component of dementia among the clients. Some with mild to moderate dementia may be helped by the administration of new medications. The introduction of cholinesterase inhibitors or NMDA receptor antagonist drugs can help individuals with dementia to improve their cognitive function slightly, although the drugs do not stop the progression of the illness.

Other clients may be admitted to behavioral health units because of mood disorders. Beyond the primary symptoms of mood disorders are issues like inertia, lack of motivation, poor nutrition, and melancholia, all of which contribute to behavioral patterns that are less than mentally enriching for clients. While this kind of mental dullness can be improved with proper treatment for the mood disorder, there is, in fact, a high co-morbidity of depression with dementia.

The cognitive stimulation programs that clients can participate in may increase alertness, attention, and perhaps stimulate more mental recall.

III. Referrals

Since everyone benefits from mental stimulation, any client may be referred to this program as long as his/her behavior is not disruptive to the group. Individuals who are disruptive may benefit from similar activities conducted in an individual session. Clients are typically assessed in behavioral health programs by completing the Mini-Mental State Exam (also known as the Folstein Scale) to determine their current cognitive function.

IV. Risk Management

There are no risks that would befall the organization from this program.

V.   Structure Criteria

This program may be offered daily in a quiet space for 45 to 60 minutes, depending on the attending skills of the group. Group size may vary, but should be small enough that all participants have frequent opportunities for responding, ideally six to eight individuals.

VI. Process Criteria

The therapist uses a variety of cognitively stimulating activities to challenge memory, retention, abstraction, and problem-solving. By keeping the mood of the group light and often humorous, clients will not feel the pressure of always having to have the right answer. The therapist may at times ask anyone in the group to respond, or at other times ask a certain individual to respond. It is important for the therapist to be aware of cognitive functioning levels so that s/he can target questions that are appropriate to the skill level of each participant. Some activities operate by taking turns, and the clients would know when their turns are coming up.

If the group is taking turns, some clients may be unable to respond with a successful answer. The therapist may then open the question to the entire group for help. The pace should move fairly quickly. Each person, then, can be challenged, but no one will feel on the spot, criticized, or diminished. Some clients may not be able to give a successful answer, but they may respond with positive affect in recognition when the answers are given.

At the beginning of each session the therapist will welcome participants and tell them that not everyone has to have the right answer, but that the purpose of the group is to have fun "exercising our brain cells." The group will begin with some easy mental challenges, then proceed to more difficult ones. At times when clients are fairly well matched, competition may be built into the activity. When the group is more varied in skill levels, competition will be de-emphasized.

The activities that can be used include trivia games, matching games, sensory stimulation, board games that require mental concentration, and large group games like *Wheel of Fortune, Jeopardy, Who Wants to be a Millionaire?, Are You Smarter than a 5th Grader?,* or *Cash Cab.* Some of these are available on the Wii system, but they may be too fast for the mental and physical reflexes of the geriatric population, depending on the participants. There are also commercially available, poster-sized crossword puzzles that a group can do together. Spelling bees or alphabet games using categories can be fun and stimulating.

At the end of the group the therapist recognizes clients for their participation and attendance.

VII. Outcome Criteria

As a result of participation in this program, the clients will:

1. Report having "fun"
2. Be able to give successful answers in the activity, or respond with positive affect when recognizing answers given by others

VIII. Credentialing

The recreational therapist will be certified by the National Council for Therapeutic Recreation Certification as a CTRS and will be knowledgeable about group process techniques.

IX. Bibliography

Alzheimer's Foundation: *How Alzheimer's drugs work.*
www.alz.org/research/science/alzheimers_disease_treatments.asp?. Retrieved 12/13/11.

American Health Assistance Foundation: *Alzheimer's risk factors and prevention.*
www.ahaf.org/alzheimers/about/risk/. Retrieved 12/13/11.

Crowe, M., Andel, R., Pederson, N. L., Johansson, B., & Gatz, M. (2003). Does participation in leisure activities lead to reduced risk of Alzheimer's disease? A prospective study of Swedish twins. *Journal of Gerontology, 58B,* 249-255.

Doidge, N. (2007). *The Brain that Changes Itself.* New York: Penguin Group.

Fitzsimmons, S. (2008). *Brain Fitness: An Instructor's Manual of 150 Exercises for People with Low to High Cognitive Function.* State College, PA: Venture Publishing.

Fitzsimmons, S. & Buettner, L. L. (2009). The recreational therapist's role in treating delirium. *American Journal of Recreation Therapy, 8*(1), 33-47.

Gediman, C. L. & Crinella, F. M. (2005). *Brainfit: 10 minutes a Day for a Sharper Mind and Memory.* Nashville, TN: Rutledge Hill Press.

Hultsch, D. F., Hertzog, C., Small, B. J., & Dixon, R. A. (1999). Use it or lose it: Engaged lifestyle as a buffer of cognitive decline in aging? *Psychology and Aging, 14*, 245-263.

Willis, S. L. & Nesselroade, C. S. (1990). Long-term effects of fluid ability training in old-old age. *Developmental Psychology, 26*, 905-910.

Wilson, R. S., Mendes de Leon, C. F., Barnes, L. L., Schneider, J. A., Bienias, J. L., & Evans, D. A. et al. (2002). Participation in cognitively stimulating activities and risk of incident Alzheimer's disease. *Journal of the American Medical Association, 287*, 742-748.

Treatment Plans

Although the appearance of treatment plans varies widely from one hospital setting to another, the content (long-term and short-term goals, behavioral objective, and discharge plans) is fairly consistent. Some facilities are excellent at completing truly interdisciplinary or integrated treatment plans. Despite requirements for regulatory agencies, some programs persist with variations of multi-disciplinary plans that allow each discipline to formulate its own treatment goals for the client. There are many hospital programs that have computerized their particular systems of treatment planning.

Individualized treatment planning is a critical step in the therapeutic process. In psychiatric settings, the process of treatment planning follows an interdisciplinary, problem-centered model. This problem-centered approach was largely recommended by the Joint Commission, which accredits psychiatric programs. In addition, this approach has been used as the model for treatment planning by state departments of mental health which license psychiatric beds and programs.

The problem-centered approach, as it is used in recreational therapy, includes the following steps:

1. An assessment of the client's psychosocial and leisure functioning
2. An identification of the client's strengths and weaknesses
3. A determination of therapeutic goal(s) or outcome(s) that the client can realistically achieve as a result of treatment
4. Behavioral objectives, or steps that are written in behavioral and measurable terms, that the client will meet in order to accomplish each goal
5. Intervention strategies that staff will use to assist the client in accomplishing the behavioral objective
6. A review date when the plan for the client will be evaluated and either continued, revised, or discontinued

The treatment plans in this book are offered to recreational therapists and students as guidelines to problem-centered, individualized treatment planning.

This collection of goals, behavioral objectives, and interventions, based on identified problems of the client, are intended for instructional use and to aid the process of standardization. By sharing common interventions, our field will be able to accumulate information that will help further measurement of the efficacy of our services.

These treatment plans, of course, are not all inclusive. There are other problems that psychiatric clients present to us and other goals and objectives that we may identify. As the line between "professional territories" continues to erode, we may also find that the types of interventions we direct may have been thought of historically as belonging to another field. Or, a professional with different training may help implement some of the services historically thought of as belonging only to recreational therapy.

While these sample treatment plans were written based on our practice with behavioral health clients, the therapist may find many of these useful with clients who have rehabilitation or general medical diagnoses as well. Difficult behaviors are not limited to the mental health setting.

To use these treatment plans, the therapist will first need to determine the type of problem that should be addressed. This portion of the book has the treatment care plans divided into five sections: behavioral, affective, cognitive, physical, and leisure. The first page of each section has a master list of the problems written up as treatment plans. Using the master list of problem-oriented plans, the recreational therapist can locate the specific treatment plan that s/he wants to review. The therapist will want to review the written treatment plan and then make modifications to that plan to make it more specific to each client's treatment needs.

Creating original and descriptive documentation on each client's status for any aspect of treatment can be challenging. At the bottom of the page you will find a short thesaurus of terms which relate to the treatment plan on that page. You can use these words to help create a more descriptive chart note or to help modify the treatment plan to match the needs of your client.

Behavioral Domain

The following treatment plans are available in the behavioral domain.

1. Resistance to Treatment
2. Poor Time Management
3. Poor Impulse Control, Violating Others' Personal Space
4. Poor Impulse Control, Walking away from Group
5. Poor Personal Hygiene
6. Anxious Behavior
7. Extreme Agitation
8. Low Tolerance for Interaction
9. Loud Voice
10. Intrusiveness
11. Demanding
12. Manipulation
13. Superficiality
14. Passivity
15. Paranoia, Distrust
16. Obnoxiousness, Offensive Behavior
17. Overt Hostility
18. Hyper-Talkative
19. Somaticizing
20. Hopelessness
21. Obsessive-Compulsive
22. Insomnia

Resistance to Treatment

Problem

Resistance to treatment

Goal

To accept treatment and make progress toward recovery.

Objective

- Client will negotiate and agree to a limited schedule to begin.
- Client will be able to explain the purpose of the therapy.
- Client will attend 50% (75%, 100%) of scheduled groups this week.
- Client will respond to activity topic 1x (2x, 3x) in group.
- Client will choose 1 (2, 3) activities each day to engage in during free time.

Intervention

- Compromise about schedule to start. Make brief daily visits to increase rapport.
- Establish a verbal/written agreement for attendance.
- Ask client to identify goals for admission and how recreational therapy can help meet these goals.
- Remind client that s/he can help in getting well by taking an interest in activities.
- Review content of group beforehand.
- Remind about groups beforehand.
- Draw client into activities on unit in free time, introduce to peers to help establish rapport.

Negative Terms To Aid Documentation

aloof	intimidating	refuses
avoids routine	intractable	reluctant
breaks rules	manipulative	resistant
challenging	menacing	territorial
condescending	mocking	tests limits
confrontational	noncompliant	testy
derogatory	opinionated	unacceptable
egocentric	oppositional	uncooperative
evasive	questions authority	unfriendly
immobile	rebellious	willful
immovable	recalcitrant	

Positive/Neutral Terms To Aid Documentation

active	helpful	reliable
agreeable	inclined	responsive
compliant	invested	successful
cooperative	motivated	willing
enthusiastic	redirectable	

Poor Time Management

Problem
Poor time management

Goal
To increase time management skills

Objective

- Client will arrive on time for group 50% (75%, 100%) of time.
- Client will review his/her schedule for the day before breakfast and again after lunch.

Intervention

- Review client's schedule of activities; ask client if there are any questions about the groups.
- Talk with client about the effect of his/her lateness on the group, and client's responsibility to follow schedule.
- Help client identify time management techniques to get organized on time.
- Remind client about scheduled groups 15 minutes before time.

Negative Terms to Aid Documentation

controlling	creates unnecessary work	dawdles
disoriented	habitual tardiness	late
loiters	overworked	postpones
procrastinates	stalls	too busy
watches clock	underestimates time	

Positive/Neutral Terms to Aid Documentation

direction	interval	regulates
duration	on time	schedule
early	organized	self-directed
handles	prompt	timely
industrious	punctual	well-timed

Poor Impulse Control, Violating Others' Personal Space

Problem

Poor impulse control, e.g., turning stereo up loudly whenever s/he wants to

Goal

To improve impulse control.

Objective

- Client will not turn volume up during activity.
- Client will ask others before doing something that intrudes on his/her space with 0 (1, 2) errors in a 24-hour period.

Intervention

- Provide client with a clear guideline of what is too loud by using the numbers on the volume control or other, similar means.
- Ask client to respect other clients in the room.
- Offer to give client the opportunity to play loud music later at a convenient time and location.
- Draw client into another activity to refocus attention.

Negative Terms to Aid Documentation

aggressive	excitable	rash
annoying	hostile	short fuse
attention-seeking	impetuous	unaware
belligerent	lashes out	uninhibited
controlling	loses control	unpredictable
distractible	poor impulse control	

Positive/Neutral Terms to Aid Documentation

aware of boundaries	redirectable	sociable
calm	respectful	tactful
cooperative	responsive	wandering
mannerly	sensitive	

Poor Impulse Control, Walking Away from Group

Problem
Poor impulse control, walking away from group

Goal
To improve impulse control.

Objective

- Client will participate in activity 10 (20, 30) minutes increasing participation time 5 minutes per group.
- Client will stand up but remain with activity.
- Client will take 5-minute break and then return to activity.

Intervention

- Ask client to try to remain another 5 (10, 15 minutes).
- Call client by name to draw client's attention back to activity.
- Allow client to take a short stretch if necessary.
- Use gross motor activity to release anxious tension.

Negative Terms to Aid Documentation

abrupt	fidgety	short attention span
anxious	impulsive	stray
AWOL	meander	uncomfortable
compelled	overstimulated	wander
drift	ramble	
eloped	roam	

Positive/Neutral Terms to Aid Documentation

attention span	focused	stationary
attentive	patient	stays with group
comfortable	planted	tolerant
concentration	redirectable	
cooperative	settled	

Poor Personal Hygiene

Problem
Poor personal hygiene

Goal
To improve self-care skills.

Objective

- Client will be dressed, groomed, and wearing shoes prior to group.
- Client will correct self-care deficiency with 1 (2, 3) verbal reminders.
- Client will be able to identify proper self-care regimen (can be broken down into individual tasks — bathing, washing hair, brushing teeth, etc.).
- Client will demonstrate ability to clean his/her own clothes.

Intervention

- Use time management strategies. Suggest to client that s/he get up a little earlier in the morning to be ready on time, suggest bringing an alarm clock from home.
- Provide client with a written or pictorial guide to appropriate dressing to be used as a checklist.
- Remind client one-half hour before group so that s/he has time to get ready.
- Discuss personal appearance as an issue of pride and self-esteem.
- Reinforce rule about appropriate dress and appearance for groups.

Negative Terms to Aid Documentation

baggy	ill-fitting	poor self-care	tight-fitting
disheveled	ineffective deodorant	poor taste	tobacco-stained
dressed to offend	matted hair	rumpled	unbuttoned
eccentric	messy	scraggly hair	unkempt
excessive perfume	neglected appearance	seductive appearance	unzipped
flashy	offensive body odor	sloppy	worn
food-stained	out of shape	slovenly	
grungy	overdressed	smelly	
heavy makeup	overlong nails	soiled	

Positive/Neutral Terms to Aid Documentation

appropriate makeup	fashionable	meticulous	tidy
careful	fresh breath	neat	well groomed
clean	good taste	shaved	

Anxious Behavior

Problem

Anxious behaviors

(fidgeting, difficulty staying in chair, tapping, purposeless actions)

Goal

To decrease anxious behaviors.

Objective

- Client will tolerate activity 5 (10, 15,...) minutes without demonstrating anxious behavior.
- Client will stop anxious behavior with 1 (2, 3) verbal reminder(s).
- Client will stop behavior with one signal cue from therapist.

Intervention

- Ask client to try activity for a certain amount of time, agree to allow client to leave the activity after the agreed upon time if s/he wishes.
- Use gross motor activities to relieve tension, e.g., exercise, sports, games.
- Identify a signal cue with client to use when the behavior is exhibited.
- Provide client with an alternative anxious behavior that is less distracting to the group (e.g., a length of cotton ribbon to fidget with instead of tapping a pencil).

Negative Terms to Aid Documentation

bothered	nervous	sitting on edge of chair
clenching hands	nonproductive movements	sweaty palms
concerned	oversensitive	tapping
excessive perspiration	overstimulated	tense
fearful	pacing	tightness in chest
fidgeting	panicking	troubled
hugging self	perturbed	uneasy
inhibited movements	racing heartbeat	vulnerable
insecure	repetitive movements	worried look
nail biting	restless	

Positive/Neutral Terms to Aid Documentation

amenable to suggestions	composed	poised
at ease	confident	quiet
calm	patient	redirectable
collected	peaceful	relaxed
comfortable	placid	

Extreme Agitation

Problem
Extreme agitation

Goal
To decrease agitation.

Objective

- Client will go to his/her room when prompted to decrease stimulation.
- Client will develop 1 (2, 3) strategies to reduce agitation.
- Client will recognize beginning of agitation and use strategies to reduce agitation 50% (75%, 100%) of the time.

Intervention

- Speak calmly to client.
- Set firm limit.
- Allow client to miss group at this time.
- Advise nursing staff on client's condition.
- When agitation is beginning, suggest to client that s/he use one of the planned strategies.

Negative Terms to Aid Documentation

aggressive	hurried	restless
angry	hyperactive	squirmish
destructive	impatient	stirred up
disturbed	inappropriate	tense
easily excitable	irritable	throwing tantrums
exaggerated	provoking	
frantic	psychomotor agitation	

Positive/Neutral Terms to Aid Documentation

calm	even-tempered	relaxed
compliant	not excitable	stable
cooperative	not rushed	steady
easy-going	quiet	subdued

Low Tolerance for Interaction

Problem

Low tolerance for interaction

Goal

To increase tolerance for interaction.

Objective

- Client will interact with therapist 5 (10, 15) minutes 1x (2x...) per day.
- Client will interact in group setting 10 (20, 30) minutes 1 (2, 3) times per day.

Intervention

- 1:1 approach. Use non-threatening, matter-of-fact approach. Use parallel activities or activities that do not require a lot of talking.
- Allow client to play or sit alone at first, or in parallel activities.
- Allow for attendance without participation.
- As tolerance improves, pair client with a peer or staff.
- Gradually draw client into small-group cooperative activities.

Negative Terms to Aid Documentation

avoidance	insecure	reluctant
disorganized	intimidated	remote
distracted	isolates self	resistive
distrustful	minimal interaction	shy
doesn't know what to say	negative	withdrawn
guarded	over-stimulated	

Positive/Neutral Terms to Aid Documentation

agreeable	endurance	reciprocal
amicable	engaged	socializes
builds rapport	friendly	sympathetic
caring	good social skills	
empathetic	initiates interaction	

Loud Voice

Problem

Loud voice

Goal

To speak in a normal tone of voice.

Objective

- Client will use normal tone of voice after 1 (2, 3) reminder(s) from staff.
- Client will identify other ways to effectively get attention besides using a loud voice.
- Client will succeed in getting needs met with alternate method.
- Client will modify loud voice behavior with just 1 (2, 3) cue(s) required from the therapist in a 30 (60) minute activity.

Intervention

- Remind client to calm down and speak slowly in a normal tone of voice.
- Suggest other ways to get attention than using a loud voice.
- Establish signal cue with client to use when behavior is exhibited.

Negative Terms to Aid Documentation

boisterous	high-pitched	screaming
controlling	labile	shrill
excessive	noisy	
harsh	overbearing	

Positive/Neutral Terms to Aid Documentation

adequate	conversational tone	pleasant
calm	inside voice	warm
composed	normal	well-modulated

Intrusiveness

Problem
Intrusiveness

Goal
To improve social skills.

Objective

- Client will interrupt conversation less than 3 (2, 1) times per 30-minute period.
- Client will respond to cueing 50% (75%, 100%) of attempts.

Intervention

- Stop activity/conversation so that client knows s/he has interrupted.
- Let client know s/he will have an opportunity to speak.
- Establish a signal cue with client to use when behavior is exhibited.
- Let client know before group what is expected from client, and ask client to monitor his/her own intrusiveness.
- Tell the client that s/he has the ability to control his/her behavior, and will be asked to leave if unable to do so.

Negative Terms to Aid Documentation

annoying	impulsive	irritating
breaking in	indifferent to social rules	manipulative
disruptive	interfering	needy
encroaching	interrupts	over-stepping
ignores boundaries	intrudes	

Positive/Neutral Terms to Aid Documentation

ability to wait	mature	takes turns
compliant	patient	tolerant
considerate	polite	
cooperative	respects boundaries	

Demanding

Problem
Frequent demanding behavior

Goal
To increase effective assertive social skills.

Objective

- Client will maintain control and wait until staff is able to assist him/her in 50% (75%, 100%) of episodes.
- Client will organize requests or demands in order of importance when requested so that the most important demands are dealt with first.
- Client will make requests or demands known in writing.

Intervention

- Tell client s/he has the right to good care but that staff are limited and unable to respond to his/her needs immediately.
- Set aside a time that is more convenient to meet with client about his/her demands or needs.
- Assist client in learning how to prioritize needs and how to identify the actual degree of urgency of each need.
- Ask client to submit requests or demands in writing.

Negative Terms to Aid Documentation

controlling	insatiable needs	socially insensitive
demanding of affection	insistent	thoughtless
demanding of favors	intimidating	wanting
disregard of others' needs	needy	
entitled	selfish	

Positive/Neutral Terms to Aid Documentation

assertive	compromises	patient
calm	flexible	waits for turn
compliant	giving	yielding

Manipulation

Problem
Staff splitting; manipulative

Goal
To eliminate staff splitting.

Objective

- Client will not play one staff against another (e.g., asking multiple staff for the same things, going to another staff person if not satisfied with the response from the first) 50% (75%, 100%) of the time.
- Client will demonstrate conflict resolution skills when feeling "wronged."

Intervention

- Redirect client back to the primary nurse or therapist to resolve the issue. Do not try to negotiate client's conflicts with other staff.
- Instruct client in basic skills of conflict resolution.
- Display conflict resolution rules in either written or pictorial form. Refer the client to these as needed.

Negative Terms to Aid Documentation

attempts to con	evasive	self-serving
controlling	maneuvering	unprincipled
deceitful	opportunistic	unscrupulous
dishonest	predatory	

Positive/Neutral Terms to Aid Documentation

accepting	engaging	redirectable
assertive	honest	socially effective
cooperative	rational	

Superficiality

Problem

Superficiality, difficulty expressing feelings

Goal

To verbalize feelings.

Objective

- Client will respond to topic when requested in 50% (75%, 100%) of groups.
- Client will make comments relative to topic in 50% (75%, 100%) of groups.
- After groups client will identify his/her response to group activity when requested by therapist.

Intervention

- Use expressive media — music, art, bibliotherapy.
- Use social skills techniques, including dyads or small group discussion.
- Be supportive, non-judgmental.
- Encourage client to talk about self, experiences, strengths.
- Let client know it is safe to share feelings.
- Confront superficial statements or joking that is inappropriate to content of discussion or activity.
- Discuss before or after the group the therapist's expectation regarding communicating feeling that is honest.

Negative Terms to Aid Documentation

bland	flat	tangential
constrained	indirect	unchanging
cursory	inexpressive	uninvolved
denial	masked	unresponsive
deflecting comment	passive	vacant
detached	restricted	withdrawn
evasive	shallow	
fake	simple	

Positive/Neutral Terms to Aid Documentation

accepting	engaging	involved
active	expressive	sincere
communicative	genuine	social intelligence
considerate of others	honest	socially aware
effective	initiating	socially capable

Passivity

Problem
Passivity, self-isolating

Goal
To increase interaction with environment.

To increase social interaction.

Objective

- Client will complete an individual activity by (date).
- Client will initiate verbal interaction 2x (3x, 5x, ...) each group.
- Client will assert his/her preferences in group activities.
- Client will select 1 (2, 3) activities to participate in for at least 10 (20, 30) minutes each day during free time.
- Client will evaluate his/her contribution to group activity or discussion when asked.
- Client will respond with positive affect 50% (75%, 100%) of the time.

Intervention

- Structure non-threatening fun activities to increase client's comfort level in socializing.
- Use social skills activities to promote interaction, e.g. paired activities, small group discussion.
- Teach assertion skills. Let client know that each person's opinion is valued. Confront non-assertive behavior.
- Make sure client is aware of choices available.
- Ask client to report his/her progress after each group so that client is actively working towards his/her goal.
- Use pet-assisted therapy.

Negative Terms to Aid Documentation

absent	inactive	secludes self
aloof	inert	submissive
compliant	insecure	uninvolved
detached	remote	unmotivated
docile	retreat	unresponsive

Positive/Neutral Terms to Aid Documentation

active	attentive	present
agreeable	eager	social
alert	enthusiastic	verbal
assertive	motivated	

Paranoia, Distrust

Problem

Paranoia, distrust

Goal

To increase level of trust.

Objective

- Client will participate in parallel group activity.
- Client will participate in trust-building group activity.

Intervention

- Use frequent, brief 1:1 contact.
- Listen to client, don't get into power struggles with client.
- Use matter-of-fact approach, make no demands.
- Offer activities for client's choice.
- Give client wider personal space margin.
- Encourage attendance even without participation from client.
- Use team initiatives to build trust.

Negative Terms to Aid Documentation

apprehension	fretful	suspicious
avoidance behavior	misgiving	unbelieving
disbelieve	panicked	worried
doubt	paranoid	

Positive/Neutral Terms to Aid Documentation

accepting	mutually respectful	sure
believable	plausible	trusting
credible	rational	
establishes rapport	reliable	

Obnoxiousness, Offensive Behavior

Problem
Obnoxious, offensive behavior

Goal
To develop socially appropriate behavior that is not offensive or intrusive on others.

Objective
- Client will alter offensive behavior with 1 (2, 3,...) request(s) from therapist.
- Client will explain how his/her behavior is detrimental to others when prompted.
- Client will use effective ways to get attention when needed 50% (75%, 100%) of the time.
- Client will demonstrate offensive behaviors no more than 2 (3, 4) times during a 60-minute group.
- Client will practice effective, socially appropriate behaviors each day.

Intervention
- Give feedback about how his/her behavior affects the group.
- Clearly define behaviors that aren't allowed and let client know the consequences. Follow through with consequences.
- Ask client what other ways s/he can get attention from the group.
- Give client positive reinforcement for socially appropriate behavior.
- Ask client to report his/her progress in using new social skills.

Negative Terms to Aid Documentation

abusive	impulsive	raw
bad taste	inappropriate	repugnant
cavalier	infringes on others	repulsive
clownish	intimidating	risqué
coarse	irresponsible	ruthless
controlling	lewd	shameless
disrespectful	lurid	suggestive
dominating	malicious	unbecoming
foul-mouthed	manipulative	uncivil
harassing	nasty	undignified
humiliating	off-color	unpleasant
immodest	offensive	vile
impolite	outlandish	violates social codes
improper	predatory	vulgar

Positive/Neutral Terms to Aid Documentation

accessible	friendly	polite
compassionate	kind	relaxed
cooperative	mannerly	respectful
dignified	mature	social

Overt Hostility

Problem
Overt hostility, angry outbursts, throwing things, threatens to harm self or others

Goal
To regain control of impulses.

Objective

- Client will regain control, will be able to discuss angry feelings without loud, aggressive outbursts.
- Client will identify 1 (2, 3) triggers of anger.
- Client will identify distortions in his/her thinking that lead to overreacting.
- Client will identify 1 (2, 3, ...) positive ways to express anger.
- Client will write in journal daily.

Intervention

- Give client space and distance. Remain calm. Let client know s/he can vent anger in a socially acceptable manner. Do not become defensive or get involved in power struggle with client. Ask client how s/he can better deal with anger.
- Let client know what the consequences are of continuing overtly hostile or aggressive behavior. Call for additional staff assistance and follow through with procedures to manage aggressive outbursts.
- When client is calmed down, ask him/her to process what has happened.
- Instruct client in principles of cognitive therapy and common distortions.
- Teach assertion skills.
- Encourage journaling.
- Provide appropriate gross motor activities and relaxation training when client is not angry.

Negative Terms to Aid Documentation

abrupt	exacerbating	indignant
animosity	exchange blows/words	lashes out
aroused	explosive	miffed
assaultive	faulty reasoning	offensive
bitter	flare-up	over-stimulated
boiling with rage	fume	provoke
bothered	grudge	rage
combative	heated	rash
dangerous	homicidal ideation	reckless
destructive	impetuous	repay

115

retaliating	takes offense	vindictive
revenge	testy	worked up
self-injurious behavior	threatening	wrath
self-mutilating	vengeful	

Positive/Neutral Terms to Aid Documentation

compliant	in control	rational
conscientious	kind	redirectable
cooperative	mannerly	respectful
dignified	mature	self-respecting
hopeful	patient	

Hyper-talkative

Problem

Pressured speech, hyper-talkativeness

Goal

To speak at normal pace.

Objective

- Client will slow down speech when directed 1x (2x, 3x).
- Client will talk in normal pace so that others can easily comprehend.
- Client will recognize when situation leads to pressured speech and use appropriate methods to reduce pressured speech without staff prompting (e.g. "I need to take a deep breath.").

Intervention

- Provide feedback to client, ask him/her to calm down and repeat what s/he has said.
- Tell client that s/he is talking non-stop.
- Establish a pre-arranged signal that staff can use with client to signal that speech is too fast.
- Suggest time out if too stimulated by activity.
- Use audio tapes or videotapes of behavior to show behavior to client.
- Provide client with guidelines on good communication/listening skills in written or pictorial format. Review with client as needed.

Negative Terms to Aid Documentation

accelerated	long-winded	slurring
babble	loquacity	stuttering
chant	monologue	too much information
chattering	non-stop	unintelligible
expansive	quickly	utter
gush	rapidly	verbose
hasty	run-together	wordy
hyper-verbal	rush	

Positive/Neutral Terms to Aid Documentation

articulate	inflection	talkative
dialogue	measured	tempo
enunciation	pace	well modulated
expressed	pronounce	

Somaticizing

Problem

Somaticizing

Goal

To decrease somaticizing.

Objective

- Client will concentrate on activity 15 (30, 60) minutes without somatic complaints.
- Client will choose level of activity that does not increase somatic complaints.
- When asked, client will prioritize somatic complaints into ones that need attention and ones that can wait.
- Client will identify healthy outlets for personal expression.
- Client will make a plan for the effective use of leisure skills to reduce attention to pain and emotional suffering.

Intervention

- Let client know s/he can participate at his/her own pace, that there are many activities, resources, roles available to him/her within the structure of the activity.
- Don't reinforce somatic complaints with discussion.
- Listen, then redirect client's attention back to activity. Use matter-of-fact approach. Refer client with somatic complaints back to nurse or physician.
- Teach assertion skills.
- Teach relaxation/meditation techniques.
- Instruct client in the co-morbid relationship of pain with depression and stress.
- Instruct client in the power of diversion from pain as a way of reducing suffering.

Negative Terms to Aid Documentation

affliction	grumbly	malady	self-centered
ailment	hypochondria	morbid thoughts	sickness
complaining	illness	obsessing	symptoms
distractible	limited attention	preoccupied	whiny

Positive/Neutral Terms to Aid Documentation

attentive	factual	honest	realistic
authentic	genuine	perception	validates
directable	healthy	rational	

Hopelessness

Problem

Discouragement, lack of hope

Goal

To have hope for recovery.

Objective

- Client will continue use of treatment program, will attend 50% (75%, 100%) of scheduled groups per day.
- Client will set personal goal for each day and report on progress.
- Client will complete task by (date).
- Client will choose 1 (2, 3) activity to pursue in free time daily and complete it.

Intervention

- Remind client that there are no miracles, that recovery takes time, and that staff will continue to work with him/her to get well.
- Ask client to consider what alternatives may help at this point, and how the staff can be helpful.
- Ask client to set a personal daily goal and identify steps needed to meet this goal. Ask client to report on progress daily.
- Use success-oriented activities.
- Help client see that what s/he does makes a difference.
- Provide client with resources to use.

Negative Terms to Aid Documentation

despair	give up	submissive
despondency	inconsolable	surrender
discouraged	pessimistic	uncomfortable
disheartened	quitting	unrealistic
dismay	ruined	useless

Positive/Neutral Terms to Aid Documentation

assured	future-oriented	optimistic
comfort	goal-oriented	positive
confident	hopeful	realistic
enthusiastic	motivated	secure

Obsessive-Compulsive

Problem
Obsessive-compulsive behavior

Goal
To increase ability to function in treatment and activities of daily living.

Objective

- Client will participate in activity 15 (30, 45, ...) minutes and not let compulsions interfere with activity performance.

Intervention

- Ask client what s/he feels out of control about and discuss ways of resuming control of impulses through recreation participation.
- Decrease emphasis on competition, perfection, and product completion, not keeping score in a game, or asking client to describe how it felt to create a drawing instead of evaluating how s/he did. Emphasize the pleasure in the process.
- Focus attention on pleasurable activities to decrease preoccupation with rituals.
- Redirect or distract client from obsessive-compulsive behavior.

Negative Terms to Aid Documentation

controlling	intense	rechecking
elaborate planning	meticulous	repetitive
excessive cleaning	over-attentive to detail	ritualistic
excessively careful	perfectionism	ruminating
hoarding	preoccupations	work-oriented

Positive/Neutral Terms to Aid Documentation

calm	easy going	process-oriented
centered	fun-loving	rational
coping	not pressured	relaxed

Insomnia

Problem
Difficulty sleeping

Goal
To get sufficient sleep at night.

Objective

- Client will sleep 6-8 hours a night.
- Client will report successful use of relaxation tapes or other interventions.
- Client will get up at appropriate time each day.
- Client will not nap during the day.
- Client will refrain from drinking caffeine after noon.
- Client will refrain from exercising within two hours of bedtime.
- Client will turn off all computer or other video screens at least one hour before bedtime.

Intervention

- Instruct client in relaxation techniques to help sleep.
- Furnish tapes and player to fall asleep with.
- Instruct client in proper sleep hygiene, getting up at regular time in the morning, maintaining an active daily schedule, eliminating napping, going to bed at the same time, not using video screens an hour before going to bed, not watching TV in the bedroom.
- Encourage gross motor exercise up to 2 hours prior to bedtime.

Negative Terms to Aid Documentation

aroused	interrupted sleep	reversal of sleep cycle
cat naps	irregular bedtime	sleep deprivation
chronic fatigue	lethargy	sleep disruptions
difficulty falling asleep	night terrors	sleepless
difficulty staying asleep	nightmares	vivid dreams
drowsy	poor sleep environment	wakefulness
early waking pattern	racing thoughts	wide-awake
insomnia	restless sleep	

Positive/Neutral Terms to Aid Documentation

calm	placid	relaxed
energized	quiet	total sleep time
effective strategies	refreshed	well-rested

121

Affective Domain

The following treatments are appropriate for the affective domain.

1. Flat Affect
2. Anhedonia
3. Inappropriate Laughter
4. Overly Bright
5. Lability
6. Low Self-Esteem
7. Anger
8. Anxiousness

Flat Affect

Problem

Flat, depressed affect

Goal

To increase appropriate expressions of affect.

Objective

- Client will express self verbally 2x (4x, 6x, ...) each group.
- Client will brighten affect within context of treatment modality.
- Client will demonstrate affect appropriate to content of activity 50% (75%, 100%) of time.
- Client will rate his/her depression on a 0-10 scale daily with an improvement noted each day.

Intervention

- Use expressive media as alternate means of expression. Engage in affect-enhancing activities such as music, reminiscence, areas in which the client has special skills, dance, social recreation, and games.
- Use humor.
- Encourage client to talk about self, his/her likes, dislikes, good times.
- Use non-judgmental, supportive approach.
- Use positive psychology techniques.

Negative Terms to Aid Documentation

absence of spontaneity	constrained	indifferent
apathetic	expressionless	inhibited
artificial	fixed affect	labile
bland	forced smile	shallow
bored	humorless	somber
cheerless	incongruous to situation	unresponsive

Positive/Neutral Terms to Aid Documentation

brightens in context	normal range	smiling
congruent affect	range of emotions	warm
face reflects emotions	relevant	

Anhedonia

Problem
Anhedonia, takes no enjoyment in activities

Goal
To increase enjoyment in normal activities.

Objective

- Client will identify activities enjoyed in past and identify what was enjoyable about them.
- Client will identify his/her barriers to enjoyment.
- Client will choose an activity and participate 15 (30, 45, ...) minutes each day.
- Client will participate in physical exercise for 15 (30, 60) minutes daily.

Intervention

- Assess client's leisure history, patterns, likes, and dislikes. Use either the Leisure Diagnostic Battery — Perceived Freedom Scale or the Leisure Satisfaction Measure to determine relevant issues. The Leisure Attitude Measurement may be helpful in identifying constraints due to attitude. Use Leisurescope Plus, Leisure Interest Measure, or other interest inventories to determine personal preferences.
- Explore leisure attitudes, values, and expectations learned at home. Discuss more useful leisure attitudes, values, and expectations to increase life satisfaction and stress management.
- Use positive psychology techniques.
- Discuss client's responses to activities and the benefits derived.

Negative Terms to Aid Documentation

apathy	emptiness	melancholy
blocked	forlorn	minimal response
callous	indifference	mirthless
cheerless	inhibited	miserable
despairing	lack of satisfaction	no interests
emotional impoverishment	low expectations	profoundly unhappy

Positive/Neutral Terms to Aid Documentation

enjoyment	in the state of flow	preferable
fun	intrinsic reward	relish
gratification	motivated	self-efficacy
happy	pleasurable	stimulated

Inappropriate Laughter

Problem

Inappropriate laughter

Goal

To laugh and use humor in appropriate ways.

Objective

- Client will demonstrate affect appropriate to content of activity 50% (75%, 100%) of time.

Intervention

- Give client feedback if laughter is inappropriate or incongruous to present activity.
- Check to see if client is hallucinating. Notify medical staff if necessary.
- Reorient client to the present situation and let the client know why his/her laughter may be incongruous.

Negative Terms to Aid Documentation

anti-social	hurtful	offensive
bizarre	illogical	psychotic
delusionally exaggerated	little insight	responding to internal stimuli
excessively boisterous	manic	uninhibited
hallucinating	odd	

Positive/Neutral Terms to Aid Documentation

amusing	genuine	relevant
comical	good sense of humor	sincere
congruent	healthy	
funny	mature	

Overly Bright

Problem
Overly bright affect

Goal
To have affect appropriate to content.

Objective

- Client will express self in a non-effusive manner in a group setting 50% (75%, 100%) of time.
- Client will share genuine feelings in a normal tone of voice and with normal affect when those feelings occur.

Intervention

- Tell client that being overly bright doesn't seem correct for this situation, that it's often a sign of being manic.
- Give client an opportunity to vent feelings in a private space.
- Speak very quietly and calmly with client.
- Use drama and other expressive modalities to practice a variety of emotions.
- Use a feelings chart or pictures to help client identify current feeling.

Negative Terms to Aid Documentation

artificial	effusive	grandiosity
covering	elated	laughing binges
cracks jokes	euphoric	unrealistic
dramatic	expansive	

Positive/Neutral Terms to Aid Documentation

appropriate affect	empathic	in touch with feelings
cheerful	genuine	realistic expressions
congruent	gregarious	relevant

Lability

Problem
Lability

Goal
To stabilize moods.

Objective

- Client will cease crying and resume activity with 1 (2, 3) cues from therapist.
- Client will describe current emotion to therapist when asked.

Intervention

- Listen to client, use light touch if a rapport has been established, ask if there is something you can do for him/her. Then ask client to identify ways of using this activity to increase positive feelings about self and to resume control.
- Refocus client's attention to activity.
- Use positive psychology techniques.
- Assist client in learning healthy coping mechanisms and problem-solving skills.

Negative Terms to Aid Documentation

abrupt change	intense	sobbing
changeable	moaning	unstable
crying	mood swings	whimpering
excessive	rapid fluctuation	

Positive/Neutral Terms to Aid Documentation

calm	even-tempered	steady
composure	regulated	temperate
control	restrained	
easy-going	stable	

Low Self-Esteem

Problem
Low self-esteem

Goal
To increase self-esteem.

Objective

- Client will successfully complete a recreation project or game.
- Client will make 1 (2, 3, ...) positive statement(s) each group.
- Client will identify 3 (5, 10) personal strengths.
- Client will provide one positive statement about self for each negative comment about self when prompted.
- Client will learn one new skill.

Intervention

- Focus on success-oriented activities within the client's ability range.
- Use initiatives.
- Give client positive feedback.
- If client does not initiate, ask for positive statement.
- Examine client's pattern of putting self down with him/her. Ask client to start a list of positive statements about self and add to it each day.
- Use positive psychology techniques.
- Help client explore ways to feel good about self.
- Teach new skills as needed.

Negative Terms to Aid Documentation

impressionable	presumes	self-image
intimidated	self-judging	self-pitying
misconception	self-blame	sensitive to criticism
overwhelmed	self-deprecating	vulnerable
personalizes	self-effacing	

Positive/Neutral Terms to Aid Documentation

accepting	hopeful	self-approval
age-appropriate	identity	self-assurance
autonomous	poise	self-efficacy
confidence	possesses ability	self-reliance
ego-enhancing	secure	success-oriented tasks

Anger

Problem
Displays anger to the wrong person or in a manner that is not helpful to himself/herself

Goal
To assertively discuss feelings of anger.

Objective

- Client will keep a reasonable tone of voice when discussing anger.
- Client will identify distortions in his/her thinking to see if anger is the best response in this situation.
- Client will regain control after an emotional outburst.
- Client will express insight about his/her anger.

Intervention

- Ask client to speak more softly so his/her ideas can be understood. Listen empathically to client. Help client choose effective ways that s/he can respond to this situation.
- Don't overreact to client's display of anger or abusive language.
- Teach cognitive-behavioral process and distortions.
- Alert additional staff for support. Suggest client go to his/her room to calm down.
- Help client see how anger can be an appropriate emotion in many situations, but outbursts often are hurtful to the self or others and are not self-respecting.
- When calmer, ask client to draw or write about his/her anger.

Negative Terms to Aid Documentation

annoyed	heated	lack of insight	overreact
cross	incensed	livid	personalizing
displaced anger	infuriated	mad	pushing your buttons
distortions	irate	misunderstanding	rage
emotional wreck	irrational	out of control	riled
fuming	jumping to conclusions	outbursts	seething

Positive/Neutral Terms to Aid Documentation

calm	cool	rational	steady
check out the facts	easy-going	respond	suitable
collected	even-tempered	self-respecting	thoughtful
composed	in control	stable	

Anxiousness

Problem

Anxiousness, indecision, trembling, non-productive movements

Goal

To decrease anxiety.

Objective

- Client will successfully complete a recreation project or game.
- Client will identify 2 (3, 4) triggers of anxiety.
- Client will state 3 strategies to decrease anxiety after discharge.
- Client will report positive outcome of using relaxation techniques.
- Client will demonstrate a more relaxed posture.

Intervention

- Focus on success-oriented activities within the client's ability range. Furnish supplies and equipment. Give client positive feedback.
- Instruct client in effective anxiety-reducing strategies.
- Teach relaxation techniques. Count respirations before and after using the technique to show the client evidence of its effectiveness.
- Use gross motor activity, a lifelong music interest, busy work like sorting objects or folding towels, or offer refreshments.
- Use gentle touch to soothe the client, a calm voice, listen and validate the client's experience in 1:1 contact.

Negative Terms to Aid Documentation

apprehensive	fretful	shaky
concerned	frightened	tense
constant movement	jittery	trembling
indecisive	nervous	uneasy
fearful	restless	worried

Positive/Neutral Terms to Aid Documentation

calm	peaceful	still
carefree	quiet	tranquil
cool	relaxed	unbothered
composed	serene	unruffled

Cognitive Domain

The following treatments are appropriate for the cognitive domain.

1. Psychomotor Retardation
2. Psychotic Thoughts
3. Ruminating Thought
4. Poor Concentration
5. Disorientation
6. Loose Associations
7. Poor Ego Boundaries
8. Poor Body Boundaries

Psychomotor Retardation

Problem
Psychomotor retardation, slow response to stimuli

Goal
To increase psychomotor activity.

Objective

- Client will respond to question within 10 (20, 30) seconds without additional cues.
- Client will participate in gross motor exercise or games 15 (30, 60) minutes daily.
- Client will increase repetitions of an exercise 20% (30%, 50%) over baseline score.

Intervention

- Maintain eye contact. State question or remark. Be quiet, wait for response.
- Take client's hand or touch arm to establish contact.
- Control environment, eliminating distractions.
- Use progressive gross-motor activity, e.g., exercise, tossing ball, dance or movement with familiar music.
- Give client direct prompts to improve performance. Use positive attitude.

Negative Terms to Aid Documentation

anergic	hesitancy	slow to process
awkward	hypoactive	slow-paced
delay	hypokinetic	stalled
dull	indecision	suspended animation
falter	inertia	tentative
gradual	listless	unproductive
halting	lumbering	

Positive/Neutral Terms to Aid Documentation

accelerated	enliven	respond
animated	quicken	tempo
answer	react	vitality
energetic	reply	

Psychotic Thoughts

Problem

Delusions, hallucinations

Goal

To increase reality functioning.

Objective

- Client will attend to task 30 (45, 60) minutes without expression of psychotic thoughts.
- Client will refocus attention to activity when instructed by therapist.
- Client will respond in a congruent manner to activity 50% (75%, 100%) of the time during a 30-minute modality.
- Client will be able to state person, place, date, and reason for admission when requested.

Intervention

- Do not negatively reinforce delusions with discussion.
- Refocus client's attention back to structured activity.
- Draw client into concrete, familiar activities to refocus attention.
- Avoid expressive media or focusing on feelings as that leads to more free association of thought.
- Give reality orientation as needed.
- Encourage reality testing from client.
- Reassure client that s/he is safe.

Negative Terms to Aid Documentation

absent	fascination	invention
absorbed	figment	magical thinking
daydreaming	flashback	misidentifies
delusions	fragmented	nonexistent
disconnected	grandiose	optical illusion
distracted	illusion	paranoid
fabricate	imagined	preoccupied
fantasy	internal stimuli	suspicious

Positive/Neutral Terms to Aid Documentation

actual	factual	real
attentive	genuine	tangible
concentrating	objective	useful
concrete	observable	
engrossed	practical	

Ruminating Thought

Problem

Obsessive, pressing, ruminating thoughts that are hard to turn off, and that keep one awake at night

Goal

To decrease ruminating thoughts.

Objective

- Client will concentrate on activity 15 (30, 45, 60) minutes.
- Client will report interference of ruminating thoughts in daily activities has decreased by 50% (75%, 100%) of the time.

Intervention

- Reassure client that s/he doesn't need to act on his/her impulses, that s/he has control of his/her behavior.
- Provide structured activities in groups and diversional activities to pursue in free time to engage attention.
- Encourage client to initiate recreational activities in free time on unit with other clients.
- Teach relaxation and thought replacement techniques. Use cognitive therapy approach to reframe thinking.

Negative Terms to Aid Documentation

absorbed in the past	intrusive	pressured
distracted	loose association	repetitive
free association	pensive	ruminating
inattentive	perfectionistic	
indecisive	preoccupied	

Positive/Neutral Terms to Aid Documentation

attentive	concentrating	in the moment
centered	focused on here and now	relaxed

Poor Concentration

Problem
Poor concentration, inattention

Goal
To increase concentration.

Objective

- Client will attend to activity 5 (10, 15, 20) minutes 1 (2, 3) times per day.
- Client will increase number of items remembered from baseline of _____ to _____ by (date).

Intervention

- Establish client's present baseline attention span and help client build up concentration by increasing increments of activity.
- Use familiar or repetitive activities.
- If client's attention wanders, encourage a 5-minute break then resume activity.
- Call client by name to refocus attention.
- Use 1:1 activities in an environment which provides few distractions.
- Use modalities which require concentration for success.

Negative Terms to Aid Documentation

apathetic	ignores	poor attending skills
brief intervals	inattentiveness	preoccupied
daydreams	lapses of concentration	selective attention
detached	needs cueing	stimulation overload
disorganized	not engaged	unaware of surroundings
distractible	not observant	
forgets easily	oblivious	

Positive/Neutral Terms to Aid Documentation

applies self	focus	notices
attentive	follows instructions	observant
concentrates	heeds	pays attention
duration	length of time	recalls
extent	listens well	watches

Disorientation

Problem

Confusion, disorientation

Goal

To increase reality orientation.

Objective

- Client will correctly identify person, place, date, and situation when asked.
- Client will follow simple 1 (2, 3)-step instructions.
- Client will locate own room in the facility.
- Client will recognize group leader and call him/her by name 50% (75%, 100%) of time.

Intervention

- Check reality orientation, reorient as needed. Act as if condition is reversible. Repeat instructions and redirect as needed.
- Provide reality orientation board prominently on the unit. Update it daily.
- Provide opportunities to find locations in facility.
- Use validation techniques to develop rapport and calm.

Negative Terms to Aid Documentation

absent-minded	hesitant	poor historian
bewildered	loss of pathfinding skills	puzzled
cognitive decline	loss of self-care skills	requires prompting
confused	lost	spotty memory
disoriented	memory deficit	unaware
distracted	misidentifies	unfamiliar
faulty recall	perplexed	
forgetful	perseverates	

Positive/Neutral Terms to Aid Documentation

acute	familiar	oriented
alert	in contact	recent memory
aware	in touch	retention
clear	keen	sharp
compensates	long-term memory	short-term memory

Loose Associations

Problem
Loose associations, flight of ideas, rambling, tangential thinking.

Goal
To increase thought organization.

Objective

- Client will respond with an answer congruent to discussion 3 out of 5x (5/5x).
- Client will attend to task 15 (30, 45) minutes without thought interruption.

Intervention

- Tell client you don't understand how what s/he is saying is connected to what was just discussed. Ask client to rephrase what s/he wants to say.
- Avoid lengthy conversations.
- Avoid expressive media because of the tendency to free associate further.
- Focus on concrete ideas and functional activities.
- Provide structured, step-by-step tasks.

Negative Terms to Aid Documentation

circular	illogical	jumbled thoughts
digress	incomprehensible	perseverating
disorganized	incongruent	rambling
drifting	irrelevant	tangential

Positive/Neutral Terms to Aid Documentation

able to restate	goal directed	pertinent
coherent	linear thought	refocus
connection	logical sequencing	relevant
consistency	orderly	sequential

Poor Ego Boundaries

Problem
Poor ego boundaries

Goal
To understand ego boundaries, awareness of others.

Objective

- Client will remain calm when another client is agitated 50% (75%, 100%) of time.
- Client will be able to state the name of another client who is having difficulty when asked.

Intervention

- Reassure client that s/he is safe, that what is happening to another client is not happening to him/her.
- Provide calming, desensitizing activities like music or tasks that require attention.
- Use calm, reassuring voice.

Negative Terms to Aid Documentation

baffled	easily threatened	role confusion
bewildered	enmeshed	self-conscious
confused	fearful	symbiotic
dependent	insecure	sympathize
easily aroused	oversensitive	uncertain about situation

Positive/Neutral Terms to Aid Documentation

apart from	independent	secure
clear-cut	limits	self
congruent	preserve	space
detach	protected	understand
disengage	relationship	
empathize	restrained	

Poor Body Boundaries

Problem

Poor body boundaries, e.g., bumping into other clients or staff, touching others

Goal

To increase client's awareness of personal boundaries.

Objective

- Client will not touch other clients.
- Client will require redirection from touching others only once (twice) per 60-minute group intervention.
- Client will successfully get attention from staff or peer without touching.
- Client will be able to stand a comfortable distance from others 50% (75%, 100%) of time.

Intervention

- Use creative movement, dance, drama, and exercise to facilitate increased awareness of self and body.
- Talk with client about other people not wanting to be touched.
- Describe other ways to get attention without touching.
- Instruct client in the need for comfort zones.

Negative Terms to Aid Documentation

brush against	collisions	touching
close	impinges upon	unacceptable
close quarters	invading	uninvited

Positive/ Neutral Terms to Aid Documentation

adequate	comfort zone	personal space
area	conscious of	proximity
adjacent	constraint	vicinity
awareness	limits	

Physical Domain

The following treatments can be used in the physical domain.

1. Psychomotor Retardation
2. Nonproductive Body Movements
3. Unsteady Gait, Uncoordinated
4. Unsteady Stance
5. Lethargy

Psychomotor Retardation

Problem
Psychomotor retardation, slow, rigid movements or non-responsiveness

Goal
To improve physical functioning.

Objective

- Client will engage in stretching exercise 10 (20, 30) minutes daily.
- Client will take daily walk 5 (10, 20) minutes with therapist 2x a day.
- Client will catch and return a ball in a simple game for 10 (20, 30) minutes.
- Client will engage in gross-motor activity as prompted 10 (15, 20) minutes.
- Client will increase reaction to perform 10% (20%, 40%) more repetitions in a ten-minute period.

Intervention

- Stress full extension, and stretching of muscles. Avoid fast, jerking movements.
- Use music to increase interest and to slowly increase tempo of performance.
- Use familiar gross motor activities such as tossing a ball, dancing.
- Use exercise, tossing ball, video games, active games like bowling or ring toss.
- Gradually increase complexity of activities.
- Leader will increase speed gradually, asking client to keep up pace.

Negative Terms to Aid Documentation

ambulation	inhibited	slow
anergic	lag behind	stiff
decelerate	lethargic	strained
delayed	listless	struggling
difficulty with task	not spontaneous	tense
dulled expression	non-responsive	with effort
inertia	restricted	

Positive/Neutral Terms to Aid Documentation

act	energized	moving
advance	greater effort	recovery
ambulate	improved	responsive
attentive	increased	restored
determined	locomotion	spontaneous
dynamics	mobility	

Nonproductive Body Movements

Problem

Anxious, nonproductive body movements

Goal

To decrease agitation.

Objective

- Client will stop anxious body movements with one prompting from staff.
- Client will participate in goal-directed gross motor activity 15 (30, 60) minutes daily.
- Client will attend to task 10 (20, 30) minutes without nonproductive movements.
- Client will engage in relaxation techniques 10 (20, 30) minutes daily.
- Client will substitute less obtrusive movement for current anxious movement when prompted.

Intervention

- Use gross-motor activities to relieve tension and other functional activities to engage attention.
- Encourage clients to talk about anxiety and useful stress reducers.
- Teach relaxation and breathing techniques when not contraindicated.
- Suggest substitute behavior, rubbing his/her leg instead of tapping noisily on table.

Negative Terms to Aid Documentation

acts out	gestures	scratching
agitated	high-strung	self-hugging
apprehensive	impulsive	swaying
can't sit still	jerky	tapping
clutching hands	jumpy	unconscious movement
constant movement	keeps moving	uneasy
distressed	low frustration tolerance	upset
disturbance	nail biting	wringing hands
excited	overwrought	writhing
fidgets	pacing	
fret	rocking	

Positive/Neutral Terms to Aid Documentation

animated	goal-directed	soothed
at ease	movement	unconcerned
at rest	not agitated	unworried
calm	productive movement	
composed	relaxed	

Unsteady Gait, Uncoordinated

Problem
Unsteady gait, poor balance, shuffling gait

Goal
To safely ambulate.

Objective

- Client will walk with assistance to/from activity without falling 100% of time.
- Client will get up and walk with assist of one each hour.
- Client will regain ability to walk unassisted without falling.

Intervention

- Walk with client, allow client to take leader's elbow or hand, if necessary.
- Restrict exercise to chair exercise or standing exercise with a chair for balance. Avoid bending over exercises or moving head to left or right quickly.
- Refer client to physical therapy for appropriate mobility aids and exercises.
- Provide activities which help client practice compensatory skills taught by other therapists.

Negative Terms to Aid Documentation

abductor lurch	difficulty with uneven surfaces	stumbles
abnormal gait	favors one side	sways
ataxic	fearful of falling	trips
awkward	instability	unstable
broad-based stance	pigeon-toed	waddles
careens	reels	wavers
clumsy	shaky	weak side
collides with objects	shuffles	
difficulty with inclines	staggers	

Positive/Neutral Terms to Aid Documentation

ambulates	footstep	stance
center of gravity	gait	steady
compensates	hip extension	strides
equilibrium	navigates	uniform steps
even	self-assured	walks

Unsteady Stance

Problem

Extreme unsteadiness, weakness, dizziness

Goal

To maintain client safety.

Objective

- Client will not fall.
- Client will learn to handle periods of dizziness or weakness so that s/he does not restrict activities more than necessary.

Intervention

- When client complains of dizziness, instruct client to sit down.
- Monitor client complaints and client balance throughout activities. Look for trends related to medication times, time of day, etc.
- If necessary, use wheelchair to escort client to and from activity.
- Notify nursing service of any new symptoms.
- Instruct client to get up from sitting or lying down position slowly to avoid hypotension.
- If arthritic joints inhibit movement, instruct client to stand in one place briefly before walking.

Negative Terms to Aid Documentation

at risk	impaired	sways
debilitated	insecure	trips
deteriorated	lightheaded	uncertain gait
dizzy	non-weight bearing	unsafe
excessive	profound	unstable
falters	severe	unsteady
fragile	shaky	vertigo
frail	staggers	

Positive/Neutral Terms to Aid Documentation

ambulation	maximum	steady
endurance	mobility	strong
firm	partial-weight bearing	transfer techniques
full-weight bearing	safe	width of gait
hip extension	stable	
kinesthesia	stance	

Lethargy

Problem

Decreased activity level, lethargy

Goal

To increase energy.

Objective

- Client will engage in physical activity 1 (2, 3) times per day for 30 (45, 60) minutes.
- Client will engage in physical activity of choice 15 (20, 30) minutes daily.

Intervention

- Use exercise, walking, running, gross-motor games, and sports.
- Encourage client to engage in former leisure interests.
- Encourage client to develop new leisure interests.

Negative Terms to Aid Documentation

abstains	diminished	not animated
apathetic	idle	passive
avoiding	inaction	reduced
curtailed	inertia	refrains
declines	listless	sluggish
decreased	minimize	vegetative

Positive/Neutral Terms to Aid Documentation

active	augments	maximizes
alert	energized	participates
amplified	engaged	responds
animated	enhanced	spontaneous
attentive	expanding	

Leisure Domain

The following treatments can be used in the leisure domain.

1. Lack of Initiative
2. Few Leisure Interests
3. Poor Compliance with Personal Recreation Goals
4. Insufficient Participation
5. Multiple Stressors
6. Overwhelmed with Responsibilities
7. Few Social Supports
8. Knowledge Deficit
9. Requires Structure

Lack of Initiative

Problem

Lack of initiative, dependence on others to plan activities

Goal

To increase initiative.

Objective

- Client will choose one activity to play during open recreation time daily.
- Client will set and meet daily goal to initiate recreation activity in free time on unit.
- Client will follow through with his/her assigned tasks in group.

Intervention

- Help client identify the recreational activities available on the unit.
- Have client choose activity, make suggestions if needed. Make sure choice has reasonable chance of success.
- Provide materials for independent use in unstructured time. Check on client's progress daily.
- Suggest client pair with another client.
- Choose group modality in which group success depends on individual follow-through such as dramatic skits or initiatives.

Negative Terms to Aid Documentation

apathetic	indifferent	restricts
dependent	lacks progress	submits
deters	not motivated	yields
gives in	passive	
inactive	procrastinates	

Positive/Neutral Terms to Aid Documentation

active	hobbyist	preferred
aims for	inclination	pursue
aspires to	increase	push forward
autonomy	interdependent	start
begins	maximizes	targets
choose	pastime	undertakes
commence	plans ahead	volition
desires	playful	

Few Leisure Interests

Problem
Few identified leisure interests

Goal
To identify leisure interests.

Objective

- Client will complete leisure interest inventory.
- Client will be able to list at least 3 (5, 7) activities that interest him/her.
- Client will identify 3 (5, 7) interests that s/he can pursue after discharge and make a plan to access them before discharge.

Intervention

- Use Leisurescope Plus, STILAP, Leisure Interest Measure, Leisure Diagnostic Battery, Leisure Assessment Inventory, or other standardized leisure interest tool.
- Use leisure education group format, using peer support and suggestions to spark interests.
- Teach new leisure skills.
- Choose activities for groups with client input and within client's skill level.
- Use 1:1 counseling to process difficult barriers.
- Assist client in the development of skills necessary to locate community-based opportunities.

Negative Terms to Aid Documentation

anhedonic	infrequent	lack of resources
apathetic	insignificant	lack of skills
dearth	lack of interest	limited selections
eliminate	lack of motivation	poverty of activities

Positive/Neutral Terms to Aid Documentation

absorbing	familiar with	perception
amusing	fascinating	playfulness
appeals	free time	recognition
appreciation	game	recreation
attention	interest	resource knowledge
comprehend	knowledgeable	spare time
discerning	learning	sport
engrossing	leisure	understand
entertaining	opportunity	well-rounded
experience	pastime	

Poor Compliance with Personal Recreation Goals

Problem

Not meeting personal recreational goals

Goal

To increase follow-through.

Objective

- Client will accomplish personal goal 50% (75%, 100%) of the time.
- Client will identify and overcome barriers which prevented him/her from accomplishing a goal for recreation by (date).

Intervention

- Use reality therapy approach. Remain non-judgmental. Ask client if s/he still wants to accomplish this goal and when s/he expects to complete it.
- Have the client identify various steps to reaching the final goal. Use these as intermediate objectives to allow practice in setting and reaching goals.
- Check on client's progress at the agreed upon time.
- Ask client what prevented him/her from accomplishing the goal. Help client problem-solve in order to achieve results. Check on client's progress at the agreed upon time.

Negative Terms to Aid Documentation

avoids	indifferent	obstruction
barriers	insincere	opposition
blocks	interest deficit	overwhelmed
competitive	isolative	passive
complications	lack of knowledge	poor compliance
compulsions	lack of resources	restraint
constraints	limits	restricted
fear	low self-esteem	self-conscious
half finishes	not committed	sporadic
hindrance	not well thought out	unrealistic

Positive/Neutral Terms to Aid Documentation

accomplishes	engages in	pleasurable activities
achievement	finish	purposeful
aims for	follow through	quality of play
ambition	fulfilled	regularly participates
amusement	genuine	satisfying leisure
attainment	good sport	social
carries through	hobby	spectator
coherence	individual	spontaneous
completion	involved with others	sport
comprehensive	pastime	target
conclusion	playful	

Insufficient Participation

Problem
Insufficient participation in personal leisure interests, lack of interest

Goal
To increase interest and participation in gratifying leisure activities.

Objective
- Client will choose one leisure interest and participate in it at least 30 minutes a day.
- Client will resume personal interest (taking walks, carpentry, singing, needle craft, etc.) while in clinical setting and participate at least 30 (45, 60) minutes daily.
- Client will make a concrete plan for the use of free time after discharge.

Intervention
- Review client's leisure participation patterns. Use "Twenty Things I Like to Do" or similar leisure education and values clarification activities.
- Review benefits client receives from preferred leisure activities.
- Help client identify present personal needs and identify how recreation can meet client's needs (for relaxation, companionship, accomplishment, self-esteem, etc.).
- Help client recognize lack of interest as a symptom of mental illness. Offer choices and material resources for client's use.
- Have client identify barriers to leisure participation, such as money, attitudes of significant others, transportation, lack of companionship.
- Help client problem-solve to overcome barriers. Ask peers in leisure education group to assist with problem-solving process.

Negative Terms to Aid Documentation

absence of	depressed	indifferent	no interest
abstains	hesitates	inertia	no follow through
apathy	inactivity	lack of incentive	unengaged
decline	inadequate	lack of initiative	wavering
deficiency	indecision	no gratification	

Positive/Neutral Terms to Aid Documentation

amusement	fulfilled	participate	satisfied
committed	gratifying	pastime	spare time
engaged	hobbyist	playful	sport
free time	initiative	recreation	sportive

151

Multiple Stressors

Problem
Multiple stressors at home or at work

Goal
To compensate for stress.

Objective

- Client will demonstrate the ability to use a leisure activity to facilitate relaxation by reporting that after the activity the perception of stress has decreased by 50% (75%, 100%).
- Client will list significant stressors.
- Client will identify his/her physical, mental, and emotional responses to stress.
- Client will learn methods and coping mechanisms to deal with significant stress.
- Client will report using stress reduction technique with positive outcome in a stressful situation.

Intervention

- Have client identify present stresses and personal needs. Have client identify recreational activities to use for stress management.
- Use enjoyable gross-motor and social activities.
- Instruct client in frequent physical, mental, and emotional responses to stress.
- Help client identify effective coping strategies.
- Teach relaxation/meditation techniques.
- Teach time management techniques.

Negative Terms to Aid Documentation

always planning	low frustration tolerance	stress intolerance
conflicts with	low amount of exercise	struggles with
detests wasting time	no time for self	tension
disengaged	obsesses	type-A personality
estranged from supports	over-schedules self	under pressure
guilt	overuse of stimulants	underestimates time
impatience	perfectionist	unnecessary deadlines
hurried	pressure	unproductive
inability to relax	restless	workaholic
inflexible	rigid	
lives with deadlines	strain	

Positive/Neutral Terms to Aid Documentation

anger management

aptitude

assertiveness

comfortable

coping ability

delayed gratification

easygoing

effective coping

escape

experience

in the moment

limits commitments

modify

rational self-talk

relaxes

resources

self-calming techniques

skills

slows down

social support system

takes time out

takes it easy

takes time for relaxation

tolerance for ambiguity

tranquil

unhurried

Overwhelmed with Responsibilities

Problem

Overwhelmed with responsibilities, no leisure time

Goal

To increase leisure participation and satisfaction.

Objective

- Client will make a plan to take 30 minutes (1, 2 hours) for self each day.
- Client will make a realistic plan with partner to have one night out each week.
- Client will identify barriers to participation in leisure.
- Client will describe a way to overcome 1 (2, 3) barriers.
- Client will redefine "responsibilities" so they become opportunities instead of a burden. (Example: caring for an infant could be an opportunity to take a class on parenting with other supportive parents.)

Intervention

- Ask client to look at "workaholic" tendencies as a means of escaping and determine relevancy of this in his/her situation. When applicable, help client identify patterns as symptomatic of adult children of alcoholics.
- Help client role play or model assertive behavior, asking other family members to share responsibilities or improving employment situation.
- Help client problem-solve for barriers such as transportation, baby-sitters, money.
- Help client find support systems to share burdens and provide support for difficult times.
- Assist client to identify cognitive distortions and reframe situation in realistic, rational thoughts.

Negative Terms to Aid Documentation

avoids	evades	overpowering
commitments	inaction	overtaxed
deluged	inundated	overwhelmed
distorted view	obligations	overworked
encumbrance	overburdened	stressed

Positive/Neutral Terms to Aid Documentation

accountability	fulfillment	pleased
alleviates	gratifies	reduction
commitments	lessen	relaxed
contentment	mitigates	relieved
control	moderation	respite
cut back	modify	responsibilities
cut down	not so serious	satisfaction
decline	obligations	sense of responsibility
decrease	overcome	spare moments
diminish	peace of mind	spare time
ease	playful	

Few Social Supports

Problem
Few social supports

Goal
To increase social supports.

Objective

- Client will initiate interaction with peers 1 (2, 3) times each group.
- Client will identify 1 (2, 3) situations where good social support would make his/her life better.
- Client will express healthy attitude about friendship.
- Client will identify 3 ways to increase social supports and make friends after discharge.

Intervention

- Structure group activities in dyads or small groups to give client opportunity to practice social skills and increase self-confidence.
- Role-play new situations to increase client's comfort level.
- Discuss ways of feeling more comfortable in social settings.
- Use cognitive therapy techniques to help client identify distortions about friendship and friendship interaction, then identify more rational responses.
- Ask client to identify "safe" places to meet new people, e.g., support groups, leisure learning classes, clubs, church activities where participants share common interests or values.

Negative Terms to Aid Documentation

avoidance	insufficient	reserved
backward	intimidates	retiring
bashful	irresponsible behaviors	retreats
clumsiness	isolates	seclusion
co-dependent behavior	keeps aloof	self-centered
control behaviors	keeps to self	self-indulgent
dates compulsively	little interest in others	shut off from
distortions	lonely	shy
excludes	lonesome	socially anxious
exploitive of others	manipulates	sole
false beliefs	promiscuous	solitude
fearful	reacts to hearsay	sporadic
immature	reclusive	teases
incapable	reluctant	thoughtless
infrequent	remote	unaffectionate

unapproachable
unrealistic

unresponsive
withdraws

Positive/Neutral Terms to Aid Documentation

accepts feedback
acquaintances
amicable
anticipates
associates with
befriends
circle of friends
classmates
clique
cohort
colleagues
common sense
companions
compliments
confidant
consensus reality
consequences

cultivates friendships
deliberate
discerning
exchanges
familiarity
family supports
friendliness
friends
give-and-take
greeting
harmony
hospitality
interpersonal behaviors
intimate
learns from experience
likable
listens

makes friends with
plans ahead
playmates
realistic social judgment
receives compliments
reconcile
refrains from gossip
roommates
schoolmates
sensitive
sociable
social circle
social performance
socially acceptable
supportive
thoughtful
trusted by others

Knowledge Deficit

Problem
Insufficient information about community resources

Goal
To increase awareness of community resources.

Objective

- Client will learn about 1 (3, 5) community resources to fit his/her needs.
- Client will make telephone calls to gather information and initiate involvement with community resources.

Intervention

- Review community resources that client can follow-up on.
- Ask client to do the investigating while in clinical setting. Offer use of telephone.
- Assist client with skills required to use phones, voice mail, and other technologies as needed.

Negative Terms to Aid Documentation

clueless	ignorant	lack of
dearth	inadequate	not enough
deficiency	insufficient	

Positive/Neutral Terms to Aid Documentation

acquire	initiate	self-learner
call	knowledge	society
clubs	learn	sports center
coach	low-cost recreation	support group
communication	need	telephone
community	outline	transportation
community center	parks department	voice mail
confidence	prepare	where to shop
describe	recount	White Pages
detail	rehearse	write
familiarize	requirements	Yellow Pages
free entertainment	scholarships	

Requires Structure

Problem

Needs structured, day activities after discharge. (Client takes insufficient initiative in using free time constructively or requires close supervision.)

Goal

To increase daily structure.

Objective

- Client will have plans for structure after discharge.

Intervention

- Identify amount of structure required and the client's ability to participate in planning.
- Work with client, family, and social service worker to set up activities such as day treatment or adult day health care.

Negative Terms to Aid Documentation

confused	impulsive	memory impaired
decreased ability	inability to perform ADLs	no insight
delusions	incapacitated	orientation problems
disoriented	incompetent	poor pathfinding skills
does not feed self	instability	relies on others
erratic	judgment impaired	thought disorder
fluctuating	labile	unpredictable
impaired judgment	may become victim	wanders

Positive/Neutral Terms to Aid Documentation

advanced ADLs	executive functioning	regular
attendant	follow through	reliable
consistency	organization	structure
control of emotions	pattern	supervision
disposition	perception of situations	understand situation
effective decisions	reality contact	

References

References

American Psychiatric Association. (2000). *Diagnostic and Statistical Manual of Mental Disorders (Fourth Edition, Text Revision)*. Washington, DC.

American Therapeutic Recreation Association. (2000). *Standards for the Practice of Therapeutic Recreation: A Self-Assessment Guide*. Alexandria, VA.

Antonucci, T. C. (1989 Social support influences on the disease process. In L. Carstensen and J. Neale (Eds.) *Mechanisms of Psychological Influence on Physical Health*. New York: Plenum Press.

Ascher-Svanum, H. & Krause, A. A. (1991). *Psychoeducational Groups for Clients with Schizophrenia: A Guide for Practitioners*. Rockville: Aspen Publications.

Baldwin, B. (1985). *It's All in Your Head: Lifestyle Management Strategies for Busy People*. Wilmington, NC: Direction Dynamics.

Banzinger, G. & Rousch, S. (1983). Nursing homes for the birds: A control-relevant intervention with bird feeders. *The Gerontologist, 23*, 527-531.

Benson, H. (1975). *Relaxation Response*. New York. Avon Books.

Benson, H., Kutz, I., & Borysenko, J. (1985). Meditation and psychotherapy: A rationale for the integration of dynamic psychotherapy, the relaxation response, and mindfulness meditation. *American Journal of Psychiatry, 142*(1) 1-8.

Benson, H. & Stuart, E. (1992). *The Wellness Book: A Comprehensive Guide to Maintaining Health and Treating Stress-Related Illness*. New York: Birch Lane Press.

Berger, B. G. (1983). Stress reduction through exercise: The mind-body connection. *Motor Skills: Theory Into Practice, 7*, 31-46.

Best-Martini, E., Weeks, M. A., & Wirth, P. (2011). *Long Term Care for Activity Professionals, Social Services Professionals, and Recreational Therapists, Sixth Ed*. Ravensdale, WA: Idyll Arbor.

Birren, J. E. & Deutchman, D. E. (1991). *Guiding Autobiography Groups for Older Adults*. Baltimore: Johns Hopkins Press.

Biswas-Diener, R. & Dean, B. (2007). *Positive Psychology Coaching: Putting the Science of Happiness to Work for Your Clients*. Hoboken, NJ: John Wiley & Sons, Inc.

Bourne, E. J. (1995). *The Anxiety and Phobia Workbook*. Oakland, CA: New Harbinger Publications.

Bullock, C. C. & Howe, C. Z. (1991). A model therapeutic recreation program for the reintegration of persons with disabilities in the community. *Therapeutic Recreation Journal, 25*(1) 7-17.

Buettner, L. (2001). *Efficacy of Prescribed Therapeutic Recreation Protocols on Falls and Injuries in Nursing Home Residents with Dementia*. Alexandria, VA: American Therapeutic Recreation Association.

Buettner, L. (2002). Falls prevention in dementia populations. *Provider, 28*(2), 41-43.

Buettner, L. L., Cummins, P., Giordano, J., Lewis, J., Lynch, C., Peruyera, G., & Siegal, J. (2008). *Recreational Therapy for the Treatment of Depression in Older Adults: A Clinical Practice Guideline*. Weston, MA: Weston Medical Publishing.

burlingame, j., & Blaschko, T. M. (2010). *Assessment Tools for Recreational Therapy and Related Fields, Fourth Edition*. Ravensdale, WA: Idyll Arbor.

Burns, D. D. (1989). *The Feeling Good Handbook*. New York: Wm. Morrow & Company, Inc.

Butler, A. C., Chapman, J. E., Forman, E. M., & Beck, A. T. (2006). The empirical status of cognitive-behavioral therapy: A review of meta-analyses. *Clinical Psychology Review, 26*, 17-31.

Carrigan, P., Collinger Jr., G. H., Benson, H., Robinson, H., Wood, L. W., Lehrer, P. M., Woolfolf, R. L., & Cole, J. W. (1980). The use of meditation-relaxation techniques for the management of stress in a working population. *Journal of Occupational Medicine, 22*(4), 221-231.

Compton, D. M. & Iso-Ahola, S. E. (Eds.) (1994). *Leisure and Mental Health*. Park City, UT: Family Development Resources, Inc.

Conti, A., Voekl, J., & McGuire, F. A. (2008). Efficacy of meaningful activities in recreational therapy on passive behaviors of older adults with dementia. *Annual in Therapeutic Recreation, 16*, 91-104.

Coyle, C. P., Kinney, W. B., Riley, B., & Shank, J. W. (1991). *Benefits of Therapeutic Recreation: A Consensus View*. Ravensdale, WA: Idyll Arbor, Inc.

Davis, M., Robbins Eshelman, E., & McKay, M. (1988). *The Relaxation and Stress Reduction Workbook, Third Edition*. Oakland: New Harbinger Publications.

Dehn, D. (1995). *Leisure Step Up*. Ravensdale, WA: Idyll Arbor, Inc.

DeVries, H. A. (1987). Tension reduction with exercise. In Wm. P. Morgan and S. E. Goldston (eds.) *Exercise and Mental Health*. Washington, DC: Hemisphere Publishing.

Dy, S., Garg, P., Nyberg, D., Dawson, P. B., Pronovost, P. J., Morlock, L., Rubin, H., & Wu, A. W. (2005). Critical pathway effectiveness: Assessing the impact of patient, hospital care, and pathway characteristics using qualitative comparative analysis. *Health Services Research, 40*, 499-516.

Eisler, R. M., Hersen, M., & Miller, P. M. (1974). Shaping components of assertive behavior with instruction and feedback. *American Journal of Psychiatry, 131*, 1344-1347.

Epperson, A., Witt, P. A., & Hitzhusen, G. (1977). *Leisure Counseling: An Aspect of Leisure Education*. Springfield: Charles C. Thomas.

Feil, N. (1993). *Validation Therapy*. Cleveland: Edward Feil Productions

Feil, N. (1993). *The Validation Breakthrough: Simple Techniques for Communicating with People with Alzheimer's-Type Dementia*. Baltimore: Health Professions Press.

Ferguson, D. D. (1991). The development of therapeutic recreation protocols through a systematic process. Unpublished paper presented at the Midwest Symposium for Therapeutic Recreation. Oconomowoc. WI.

Ferguson, D. D. (1994). Developing protocols for leisure problems in mental health. In D. A. Compton and S. E. Iso-Ahola (Eds.). *Leisure and Mental Health*. Park City, UT: Family Development Resources, Inc.

Gabor, D. (1983). *How to Start a Conversation and Make Friends*. New York: Simon and Schuster.

Gallo, J. J., Reichel, W., & Andersen, L. (1988). *Handbook of Geriatric Assessment*. Rockville: Aspen Publications.

Gregory, B. M. (No date). CBT Skills Workbook: Practical Exercises and Worksheets to Promote Change. Eau Claire, WI: Premier Education Solutions.

Greist, J. H., Klein, M. H., Eischens, R. R., Gurman, A. S., & Morgan, W. P. (1979). Running as a treatment for depression. *Comprehensive Psychiatry, 20*, 41-54.

Grossman, A. H. (1976). Power of activity in a treatment setting. *Therapeutic Recreation Journal, 10*(4), 119-124.

Hawkins, B. (2002). *Leisure Assessment Inventory*. Ravensdale, WA: Idyll Arbor, Inc.

Hipp, E. (1985). *Fighting Invisible Tigers: A Stress Management Guide for Teens*. Minneapolis: Free Spirit Publishing.

Hipp, E. (1987). *A Teacher's Guide to Fighting Invisible Tigers: A 12 Part Course in Lifeskills Development*. Minneapolis: Free Spirit Publishing.

Hurley, O. (1988). *Safe Therapeutic Exercise for the Frail Elderly: An Introduction*. Albany, NY: The Center for the Study of Aging.

Huss, D. B. & Baer, R. A. (2007). Acceptance and change: The integration of mindfulness-based cognitive therapy into ongoing dialectical behavior therapy in a case of borderline personality disorder with depression. *Clinical Case Studies, 6*(1), 17-33.

Kane, R. & Kane, R. (1981). *Assessing the Elderly, A Practical Guide to Measurement*. Lexington: Lexington Books.

Kaufman, G. & Raphael, L. (1990). *Stick Up for Yourself! Every Kid's Guide to Personal Power and Positive Self-Esteem*. Minneapolis: Free Spirit Publishing.

Kaufman, G. & Raphael, L. (1991). *Teacher's Guide to Stick Up for Yourself! A 10 Part Course In Self-Esteem and Assertiveness for Kids*. Minneapolis: Free Spirit Publishing.

Kemp, B. (1990). *Geriatric Rehabilitation*. Boston: College-Hill Press.

Keogh-Hoss, M. A. (1994). *Therapeutic Recreation Activity Assessment*. Ravensdale, WA: Idyll Arbor.

Kloseck, M. & Crilly, R. (1997). *Leisure Competence Measure*. London, Ontario: Leisure Competence Measure Data System.

Knight, L. & Johnson, D. (1991). Therapeutic recreation protocols: Client problem centered approach. In R. Riley (ed.). *Quality Management: Applications for Therapeutic Recreation*. State College, PA: Venture Publishing, Inc.

Korb, K. L., Azok, S. D., & Leutenberg, E. A. (1992). *SEALS + Plus: Self-Esteem and Life Skills: Reproducible Activity-Based Handouts Created for Teachers and Counselors*. Beachwood, OH: Wellness Reproductions.

Leahy, R. L. (2003). *Cognitive Therapy Techniques: A Practitioner's Guide*. New York: Guilford Press.

Leavy, R. L. (1983). Social support and psychological disorder. *Journal of Community Psychology, 11*, 3-21.

Liberman, R. P., Lillie, F. J., Falloon, I. R. H., Harpin, E. J., Hutchison, W., & Stout, B. A. (1984). Social skills training for relapsing schizophrenics: An experimental analysis. *Behavioral Modification, 8*, 155-179.

Martinsen, E. W., Medhus, A., & Sandvik, L. (1984). The effect of aerobic exercise on depression: A controlled study. Unpublished manuscript.

Matheny, K. S., Aycock, D. W., Pugh, J., Curlette, W. L., Silva Cannella, K. A. (1986). Stress coping: A qualitative and quantitative synthesis and implications for treatment. *The Counseling Psychologist, 14*(4) 499-549.

McGlynn, G. (1987). *Dynamics of Fitness: A Practical Approach*. Dubuque, IA: Wm. C. Brown.

Morgan, W. P. & Goldston, S. E. (1987). *Exercise and Mental Health*. Washington, DC: Hemisphere Publishing.

Olsson, R. H. Jr. (1990). *Recreational Therapy Protocol Design: A Systems Approach to Treatment Evaluation*. Toledo, OH: International Leisure Press.

Parker, S. D. & Will, C. (1993). *Activities for the Elderly Volume 2: A Guide to Working with Residents with Significant Physical and Cognitive Disabilities*. Ravensdale, WA: Idyll Arbor, Inc.

Peterson, C. (2006). *A Primer in Positive Psychology*. New York: Oxford University Press, Inc.

Russoniello, C. V. (1991). An exploratory study of physiological and psychological changes in alcoholic clients after recreation therapy treatments. Paper presented at the Benefits of Therapeutic Recreation in Rehabilitation Conference, Lafayette Hill, PA.

Scogin, F. & Prohaska, M. (1993). *Aiding Older Adults with Memory Complaints*. Sarasota: Professional Resource Press.

Searle, M. S. & Mahon, M. J. (1993). The effects of a leisure education program on selected social-psychological variables: A three month follow-up investigation. *Therapeutic Recreation Journal, 27*(1), 9-21.

Segal, Z. V., Williams, J. M. G., & Teasdale, J. D. (2002). *Mindfulness-based Cognitive Therapy for Depression*. New York: Guilford Press.

Shary, J. & Iso-Ahola, S. (1989). Effects of a control relevant intervention program on nursing home residents' perceived competence and self-esteem. *Therapeutic Recreation Journal, 23*, 7-16.

Sime, W. E. (1987). Exercise in the treatment and prevention of depression. In W. P. Morgan and S. E. Goddamn (Eds.) *Exercise and Mental Health*. Washington, DC: Hemisphere Publishing.

Skalko, T. K. (1982). The effects of leisure education program on the perceived leisure well-being of psychiatrically impaired active army personnel. Unpublished doctoral dissertation. College Park, MD: University of Maryland.

Smith-Marker, C. G. (1988). *Setting Standards for Professional Nursing: The Marker Model*. Baltimore: Resource Applications.

Stumbo, N. J. & Wardlaw, B. (2011). *Facilitation of Therapeutic Recreation Services*. State College, PA: Venture Publishing.

Tortosa-Martinez, J., Zoerink, D. A., & Yoder, D. G. (2011). The benefits of therapeutic recreation experiences for people with Alzheimer's disease. *Annual in Therapeutic Recreation, 19*, 52-64.

Turner, R. J. (1981). Social support as a contingency in psychological well-being. *Journal of Health and Social Behavior, 22*, 357-367.

Wassman, K. B. & Iso-Ahola, S. E. (1985). The relationship between recreation participation and depression in psychiatric clients. *Therapeutic Recreation Journal, 19*(3), 63-70.

Williams, M., Teasdale, J., Segal, Z., & Kabat-Zinn, J. (2007). *The Mindful Way through Depression: Freeing Yourself from Chronic Unhappiness*. New York: Guilford Press.

Winnick, J. P. (Ed.) (1990). *Adapted Physical Education and Sport*. Champaign: Human Kinetics Books.

Wittals, H. & Greisman, J. (1971). *The Clear and Simple Thesaurus Dictionary*. New York: Grosset and Dunlap, Publishers.

Wong, S. E., Terranova, M. D., Bowen, L., et al. (1987). Providing independent recreational activities to reduce stereotypic vocalization in chronic schizophrenics. *Journal of Applied Behavior Analysis, 20*, 77-81.

Wong, S. E., Terranova, M. D., Marshall, B. D., Banzett, L. K., & Liberman, R. P. (1983). Reducing bizarre stereotypic behavior in chronic psychiatric clients: Effects of supervised and independent recreational activities. Presented at the Ninth Annual Convention of the Association of Behavior Analysis, Milwaukee, WI.

Young, J. E. (1986). A cognitive-behavioral approach to friendship disorders. In V. J. Derlego and B. A. Winstead. *Friendship in Social Interaction*. New York: Springer-Verlag.

Young, J. E. & Klosko, J. S. (1993). *Reinventing Your Life: The Breakthrough Program to End Negative Behavior and Feel Great Again.* New York: Plume Books.

Young, J. E., Klosko, J. S., & Weishaar, M. E. (2003). *Schema Therapy: A Practitioner's Guide.* New York: Guilford Press.

Zgola, J. M. (1987). *Doing Things: A Guide to Programming Activities for Persons with Alzheimer's Disease and Related Disorders.* Baltimore: Johns Hopkins Press.

Zimbardo, P. (1977). *Shyness: What It Is. What to Do About It.* Reading, MA: Wesley Publishing Company.

About the Authors

This book, *Behavioral Health Protocols and Treatment Plans for Recreational Therapy*, has evolved from the vision of Karen Grote through her more than thirty years of practice in the field, mostly in behavioral health settings. Since earning her master's degree from the University of North Carolina at Chapel Hill, Karen has worked to develop the profession as a therapist, supervisor, educator, and as a mentor. Her commitment to recreational therapy has led her to accept elected offices at the local, state, and national levels. She was one of the earlier presidents of the American Therapeutic Recreation Association, serving in FY 1991. In recent years Karen has concentrated her efforts on guiding the establishment of the Recreational Therapy Foundation by acting as its president.

Behavioral Health Protocols and Treatment Plans for Recreational Therapy marks Sara Warner's first published work in the field. Sara possesses an undergraduate degree in science with a focus in recreational therapy, as well as a master of art degree from the University of Toledo. In addition, she's been a member of the Cincinnati Dayton Area Recreation Therapy Association since 2007, where she also served on the board for two consecutive years. Sara's current professional involvement includes her full-time role as the Recreation Coordinator for the Children's Home of Northern Kentucky and part-time employment with St. Elizabeth Hospital where she serves as a recreational therapist. Cosmo, Sara's English Mastiff, also shares a love for recreational therapy and is a certified therapy dog through Therapy Dogs International (TDI).